ZERO-POINT WEIGHT LOSS

COOKBOOK FOR BEGINNERS

Eat Deliciously, Shed pounds & Stress-Free Recipes without Counting Calories for a Healthier Lifestyle.

2025

JOSE I. CONNELLY

COPYRIGHT ©

JOSE I. CONNELLY

DISCLAIMER

TABLE OF CONTENTS

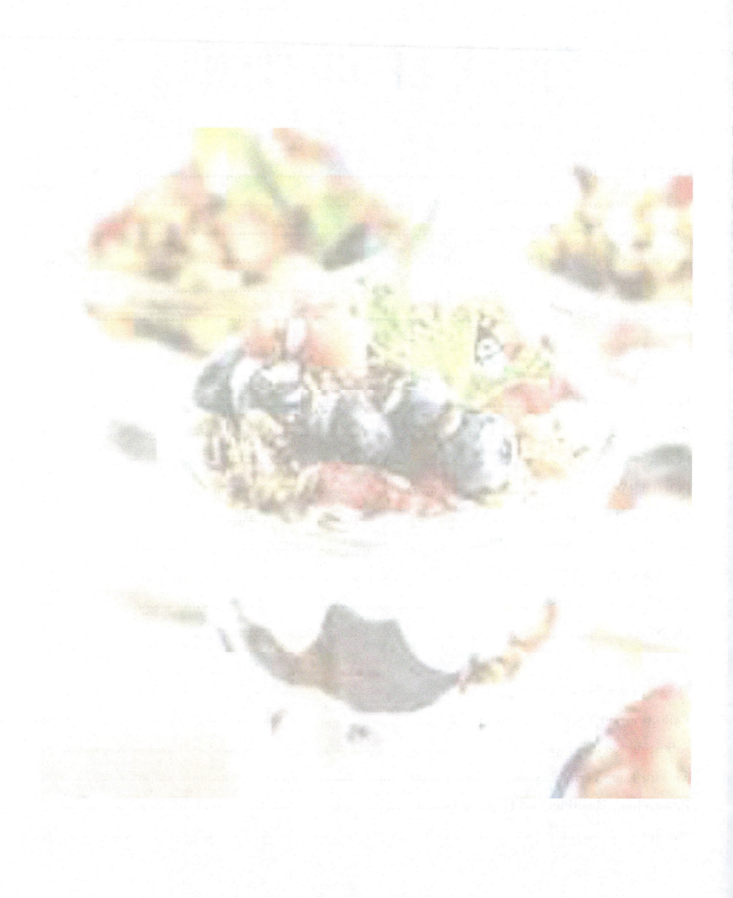

INTRODUCTION

Welcome to Zero Point Lifestyle

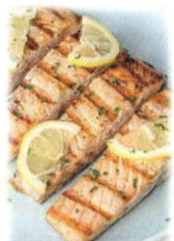

Welcome to the Zero Point Lifestyle, a new eating plan that makes weight reduction and healthy living easy, pleasurable, and long-term. This lifestyle does not include tight diets, compulsive calorie tracking, or feelings of deprivation. Instead, it's based on a strong idea: concentrating on zero-point meals.

WHAT IS A ZERO POINT LIFESTYLE?

Some meals are so low in calories and high in nutrients that they automatically help you achieve your health and weight reduction objectives, according to the Zero Point Lifestyle. These foods are filling, nutritious, and simple to integrate into your diet without worrying about portion sizes or overindulging. They contain a wide range of vegetables, lean meats, fruits, and legumes, all of which may be consumed freely.

WHY SELECT ZERO POINT?

Many diets fail because they are too difficult, excessively restricted or simply do not fit into everyday living. The Zero Point Lifestyle is unique. It enables you to enjoy tasty meals, try new recipes, and eat until you're full—all while keeping on track with your health objectives.

Here are a few reasons why the Zero Point Lifestyle is ideal for beginners:

- **No Need to Count or Track:** Forget about calculating calories, monitoring macros, or measuring each item. Zero-point items allow you to enjoy meals without having to constantly calculate.
- **Satisfying and Sustainable:** The emphasis is on nutrient-dense meals that keep you full, making it simpler to avoid unhealthy snacking and binge eating.
- **Simple and Flexible:** Whether you're cooking for yourself, your family, or guests, these recipes are simple to make and can be tailored to your preferences.

WHAT YOU CAN EXPECT FROM THIS COOKBOOK
this cookbook is meant to help you through the Zero Point Lifestyle, including:

- **Recipes That Are Delicious and Simple to Follow:** Each meal has fresh, healthful ingredients and is designed to fit smoothly into your hectic schedule.
- **A 30-Day Meal Plan:** This organized plan provides you a head start by guiding you through the lifestyle one meal at a time.
- **Tips for Long-Term Success:** Discover simple tactics for meal planning, grocery shopping, and maintaining consistency even when life becomes hectic.

YOU'RE PATH TO WELLNESS AND HAPPINESS

The Zero Point Lifestyle is more than simply a diet; it's a long-term commitment to nurturing your body and becoming a healthier, happier version of yourself. You'll see that losing weight does not have to include giving up your favorite foods or spending hours in the kitchen.

Prepare to discover a world of delectable, zero-point dishes, as well as a new way of life that is both stress-free and rewarding. Welcome to the Zero Point Lifestyle—your route to health, simplicity, and long-term success!

Let us get started!

Understanding Zero Point Foods

Zero-point foods are the basis of the Zero Point Lifestyle. These foods have been carefully chosen for their potential to fuel your body, keep you satisfied, and support your weight loss or maintenance goals—all without the need for calorie tracking or portion management. But what precisely qualifies a food as "zero-point," and how can you include these items into your everyday diet? Let's dig in.

WHAT IS ZERO-POINT FOODS?

Zero-point meals are inherently low in calories, high in key nutrients, and have no effect on your overall energy consumption. They are usually entire, unadulterated meals that your body can absorb properly. These foods promote a healthy diet by stressing fresh, healthful ingredients.

ZERO-POINT FOOD CATEGORY LIST

Here's a breakdown of the typical types of zero-point foods:

➢ **Vegetables**
   Examples include spinach, kale, broccoli, carrots, zucchini, bell peppers, and tomatoes.
   Benefits: High in vitamins, minerals, fiber, and antioxidants. They give depth and texture to dishes while remaining low in calories.

➢ **Fruits**
   Examples include apples, berries, oranges, bananas, and melons.
   Advantages: High in natural sugars for energy, vitamins, fiber, and hydration.

➢ **Lean Proteins**
   Examples include skinless chicken breast, turkey, eggs, tofu, and plain nonfat yogurt.
   Benefits: Helps with muscle repair and development while keeping you full for longer.

➢ **Legumes & Beans**
   Examples include lentils, black beans, chickpeas, and kidney beans.
   Benefits: Packed with plant-based protein, fiber, and slow-digesting carbohydrates for long-lasting energy.

➢ **Seafood**
   Examples include salmon, tuna, shrimp, and cod.
   Benefits: Rich in omega-3 fatty acids, protein, and vital minerals.

WHY ZERO-POINT FOODS ARE IMPORTANT

➢ **Promote Fullness:** These meals are high in fiber and water, so they keep you full without making you overeat.
➢ **Encourage Healthy Eating Habits:** They naturally lead you to entire, nutrient-dense foods.
➢ **Flexible and Versatile:** You may combine zero-point items in limitless combinations to make meals that suit your preferences and lifestyle.
➢ **Guilt-Free Eating:** Because these meals are low in calories, you may indulge without worrying about portion management.

HOW TO USE ZERO POINT FOODS

➢ **Base Your Meals Around Them:** Begin each meal with zero-point items. For example, make a salad with lush greens, grilled chicken, and fresh vegetables, then add a modest bit of dressing or cheese for taste.
➢ **Snack Smart:** Replace processed snacks with fresh fruits, raw vegetables, or hard-boiled eggs.
➢ **Increase Variety:** Experiment with new zero-point items to make your meals interesting and unique.
➢ **Cook Creatively:** Enhance the natural tastes of zero-point ingredients using herbs, spices, and cooking methods such as grilling, roasting, and steaming.

COMMON MYTHS ABOUT ZERO-POINT FOODS

➢ **I Can Eat Unlimited Quantities without Gaining Weight:** While zero-point items are low in calories, it is still crucial to respond to your body's hunger signals.
➢ **They're Boring or Bland**: On the contrary, zero-point meals are extremely adaptable and, with proper preparation, may be transformed into savory, gratifying dinners.

THE BALANCED APPROACH

while zero-point items are the foundation of the Zero Point Lifestyle, they are most effective when combined with a well-rounded diet. For maximum health and happiness, combine them with tiny amounts of healthy fats, whole grains, and other nutrient-dense products.

Understanding and loving zero-point meals is the secret to uncomplicated, guilt-free eating that helps you achieve your objectives. It's not about limitations; it's about plenty, sustenance, and freedom.

Are you ready to start preparing excellent meals using zero-point foods? Let's discuss how to make them the star of your meal!

Advantages of the Zero-Point Approach

The Zero-Point Approach is more than just a diet; it is a sustainable and empowering way of life. Focusing on zero-point foods simplifies your relationship with eating while providing various physical, emotional, and practical advantages. Here's how adopting this technique may improve your health and well-being.

SIMPLIFIED MEAL PLAN
One of the most notable benefits of the Zero-Point Approach is its simplicity. Meal planning becomes easier and less stressful when you don't have to calculate calories or measure each piece. You may make meals by mixing zero-point ingredients in an infinite number of combinations, allowing you complete flexibility and freedom in the kitchen.

ENCOURAGES NUTRIENT-DENSE EATING
Zero-point meals are naturally high in key elements, including vitamins, minerals, fiber, and antioxidants. By preparing your meals with these healthful components, you provide your body with the nutrition it requires to flourish while avoiding processed and calorie-dense foods.

PROMOTES FULLNESS AND SATISFACTION
Many zero-point items, including vegetables, fruits, and lean meats, are high in fiber and water. These characteristics keep you feeling fuller for longer, minimizing your chances of overeating or reaching for harmful foods. As a consequence, you may efficiently regulate hunger while eating a balanced diet.

SUPPORTS LONG-TERM WEIGHT LOSS
The Zero-Point Approach eliminates the need for restrictive diets, which makes it simpler to stick to your weight reduction goals. Instead of focusing on what you can't consume, this strategy stresses what you can enjoy, resulting in long-term habits.

REDUCES STRESS OVER FOOD
Constant calorie counting, weighing, and tracking might be taxing. The Zero-Point Approach alleviates most of the mental stress by simplifying your options. With so many zero-point dishes to choose from, you can enjoy your meals without worrying about the numbers.

PROMOTES CREATIVITY IN THE KITCHEN
The Zero-Point Approach encourages you to explore with fresh, natural ingredients. You will learn new methods to prepare and combine foods, resulting in unique meals that are both healthful and tasty. This diversity makes your diet more fascinating and pleasurable.

SUITABLE FOR ANY LIFESTYLE
Whether you're cooking for yourself, your family, or entertaining guests, the Zero-Point Approach fits into any lifestyle. It caters to hectic schedules with quick, uncomplicated dishes and provides enough diversity to satisfy diverse tastes and dietary needs.

PROMOTES LONG-TERM HEALTH

The Zero-Point Approach, which prioritizes complete, nutrient-dense meals, can help reduce the risk of chronic illnesses such as heart disease, diabetes, and obesity. It encourages healthy practices that improve overall well-being, making it an excellent option for anybody wishing to invest in their health.

PROMOTES A POSITIVE RELATIONSHIP WITH FOOD

Instead of categorizing meals as "good" or "bad," the Zero-Point Approach emphasizes abundance and balance. This perspective promotes a healthy connection with food, transforming eating into a source of sustenance and joy rather than stress or guilt.

THERE IS NO DEPRIVATION, ONLY FREEDOM

Unlike restrictive diets that make you feel deprived, the Zero-Point Approach allows you to eat large amounts of enjoyable foods. Knowing you can eat anything from an approved list of zero-point items gives you a sense of freedom and control over your eating habits.

IN SUMMARY

The Zero-Point Approach is a new, sustainable way to eat that emphasizes health, simplicity, and happiness. It's not about rules or limits, but about eating things that naturally help you achieve your goals. This strategy allows you to enjoy tasty meals, attain your target weight, and live an enjoyable and satisfying lifestyle.

Are you ready to see how this method may transform the way you eat and live? Let's get into the recipes and strategies that make the Zero-Point Lifestyle so successful and delightful!

How to Use This Cookbook

Welcome to the complete guide to the Zero Point Lifestyle! This cookbook is intended to help you adopt a healthy, stress-free way of eating without the need to monitor calories. It's full of easy, delicious recipes and useful advice to help you on your path to improved health. Here's how to make the best of it:

BEGIN WITH THE BASICS
before digging into the recipes; spend some time familiarizing yourself with the foundations of the Zero Point Lifestyle:

➢ **Understanding Zero-Point Foods:** These are the foundation of this lifestyle. Return to the previous section on zero-point meals to discover what they are and why they are useful.
➢ **Identify Your Goals:** This cookbook gives tools to help you lose weight, maintain a healthy weight, or just improve your diet.

IMPLEMENT THE 30-DAY MEAL PLAN

➢ If you are new to the Zero Point Lifestyle, the 30-day meal plan contained in this book is an excellent place to start. It's a pre-designed blueprint to assist you.
➢ Make a smooth transition to the lifestyle.
➢ Learn how to include zero-point items in each meal.
➢ Experiment with dishes that are quick, simple, and family-friendly.

➢ Use the meal plan as a guide, but feel free to combine dishes based on your tastes.

DISCOVER RECIPES

➢ This cookbook is divided into sections for simple navigation, which include:
➢ Breakfast - Fish and seafood
➢ Beef, pork, and lamb - Poultry - Vegetable sides
➢ Vegetarian mains - Snacks and appetizers - Stews and poultry
➢ Desserts

Each category has five curated recipes to accommodate a wide range of tastes and situations. Navigate to the department you're interested in and enjoy discovering foods that fit neatly into the Zero Point Lifestyle.

REFER TO THE RECIPE DETAILS
each recipe contains:

➢ **Prep and Cook Times:** Plan your meals based on your schedule.
➢ **Serving Sizes:** Scale recipes up or down to meet your requirements.
➢ **Ingredients:** Use fresh, complete ingredients.
➢ **Directions:** Cooking is simplified with clear, step-by-step directions.

➢ **Nutritional Benefits:** Discover how each cuisine promotes your health.

CUSTOMIZE RECIPES TO YOUR TASTE
The Zero Point Lifestyle is adaptable; therefore, do not hesitate to:

➢ **Swap ingredients:** Replace these products with your favorite zero-point foods.
➢ **Adjust the portions:** Scale recipes for individual dinners or large groups.
➢ **Experiment:** Add spices, herbs, or seasonings to your liking.

OFFER SNACKS AND APPETIZERS
snacking is a way of life! The snacks and appetizers area provides imaginative, healthful alternatives to keep you satiated in between meals. These are ideal for hectic days or hosting visitors.

PLAN AHEAD FOR MEAL PREP
preparing meals is essential for maintaining consistency. This cookbook can help you plan your weekly menu and prepare dishes in advance. Many meals may be frozen or reheated quickly, making your lifestyle even handier.

TRACK YOUR PROGRESS
this cookbook is a transformational tool, not merely a collection of recipes. Keep track of new recipes you've tried and enjoyed.

➢ Changes in energy levels and overall well-being.
➢ Progress toward your weight-loss or health objectives.

STAY INSPIRED
If you ever feel stuck, go back to the beginning, advice, or even the end of this book for inspiration. The meals and lifestyle changes are intended to be pleasurable, not restrictive.

MAKE IT YOURS
finally, this cookbook is a guide. Feel free to customize it by changing the recipes, making your own meal plans, or developing variants on the foods. The Zero Point Lifestyle emphasizes independence, simplicity, and happiness.

Following these steps will put you on track to mastering the Zero Point Lifestyle and enjoying the road to a healthier, happier self. Let's get cooking!

Your 30-Day Meal Plan: A Brief Overview

A detailed strategy makes it simpler to embark on a new lifestyle. This 30-day meal plan is intended to introduce you to the Zero Point Lifestyle in a planned and reasonable way. It offers a range of tasty, zero-point recipes that can help you gain confidence in the kitchen, enjoy good cuisine, and meet your health objectives.

Here's a brief summary of what to expect:

HOW THE PLAN WORKS

➢ **Balanced Approach**: Each day consists of three meals and optional snacks, with an emphasis on zero-point items and the occasional inclusion of healthy fats, grains, or dairy to keep your meals balanced.
➢ **Flexibility:** You can follow the plan as provided or customize meals to your tastes. The idea is to make healthy eating fun while also reducing stress.
➢ **Simple Recipes:** Most meals take minimum preparation, making it simple to stick to the plan even on hectic days.

WEEKLY STRUCTURE

Week 1: Get Started

➢ To ease into the Zero Point Lifestyle, stick with easy meals that use familiar products.
➢ **Breakfast:** Berry Blast Smoothie Bowl or Vegetable-Packed Breakfast Scramble.
➢ **Lunch options:** include shrimp and avocado lettuce wraps or grilled chicken salad.
➢ **Dinner options:** include zero-point beef stir-fry or lentil and spinach curry.
➢ **Snacks:** include spicy roasted chickpeas and deviled eggs with a twist.

Week 2: Exploring Variety.

➢ Introduce fresh flavors and combinations to keep meals interesting.
➢ **Breakfast options**: include overnight chia seed pudding or spinach and mushroom egg muffins.
➢ **Lunch options:** include spicy tuna cucumber bites or zucchini noodles with tomato basil sauce.
➢ **Dinner options:** include herb-crusted lamb chops or grilled portobello mushroom "steaks."
➢ **Snacks:** include mini caprese skewers and Greek yogurt dip with vegetables.

Week 3: Meal Preparation Made Easy

➢ Concentrate on dishes that are ideal for meal prep and reheating.
➢ **Breakfast options:** include zucchini and sweet potato hash or balsamic-glazed chicken thighs.
➢ **Lunch:** Classic Beef and Tomato Stew or Mediterranean Grilled Vegetable Platter.
➢ **Dinner options:** include coconut lime shrimp soup or sweet potato and black bean tacos.

➢ Snacks include cucumber and hummus roll-ups or spiced pumpkin soup.

Week 4: Increasing Confidence

➢ By this stage, you'll be more at ease with the Zero Stage Lifestyle. This week, we urge you to mix and combine your favorite dishes or try something new from the cookbook.
➢ **Breakfast:** Choose any from the previous weeks.
➢ **Lunch options:** include zero-point pulled pork lettuce wraps or stuffed bell peppers with quinoa and chickpeas.
➢ **Dinner:** Lemon Garlic Grilled Salmon or Slow-Cooked Beef with Sweet Potato Chili.
➢ Snacks include lemon and coconut energy balls or chocolate-dipped strawberries.

SUCCESS TIPS

Plan ahead

➢ Prepare by reviewing the week's meals and shopping for items ahead of time. This saves time and alleviates stress on hectic days.
➢ **Prep in Batches:** Make bigger servings of meals, such as soups, stews, or casseroles, to have leftovers throughout the week.
➢ **Listen to Your Body:** Adjust portion sizes and meal times based on your appetite and energy levels.
➢ **Stay Hydrated:** Drink enough water throughout the day for better digestion and health.
➢ **Celebrate Progress:** Note how your energy, mood, and behaviors improve as you keep to your strategy.

YOUR ZERO-POINT JOURNEY BEGINS HERE

This 30-day meal plan is your guide to living a sustainable and happy lifestyle. It's not about perfection but about growth. By concentrating on zero-point foods and implementing these recipes into your daily routine, you will set yourself up for long-term success.

Are you ready to plunge in? Let's look at the wonderful meals that will help you transform!

CHAPTER ONE

BREAKFAST

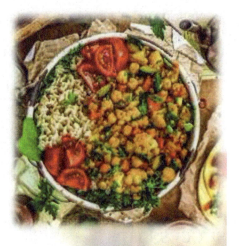

Veggie-Packed Breakfast Scramble

Prep Time: 5 minutes.

Cooking Time: 10 minutes

Total Time: 15 minutes.
Servings: 2

Points per Recipe: 0 (zero points)

Ingredients:

- 4 big eggs (or egg whites for a lower-calorie option)
- 1/2 cup sliced bell pepper (red, green, or yellow)
- Add 1/2 cup sliced onion, 1/2 cup chopped spinach, and 1/4 cup diced tomatoes.
- Add 1/4 cup chopped zucchini and 1/4 cup sliced mushrooms.
- 1 tablespoon olive oil or cooking spray (optional when sautéing)
- Add salt and pepper to taste.
- Fresh herbs to garnish (optional, such as parsley or chives)

Directions:

1. Prepare the Vegetables: Wash and cut the bell peppers, onions, spinach, tomatoes, zucchini, and mushrooms. Set aside.

2. To sauté vegetables, heat olive oil (or cooking spray) in a medium pan over medium heat. Combine the bell pepper, onion, zucchini, and mushrooms. Sauté for 4-5 minutes, until softened and gently browned.

3. Stir in spinach and tomatoes. Cook for a further 1-2 minutes, until the spinach has wilted.

4. Scramble the Eggs: In a small dish, mix together eggs, salt, and pepper. Pour the eggs into the skillet alongside the vegetables. Let them simmer for 3-4 minutes, stirring gently to scramble. Cook the eggs until completely set but still wet.

5. Serve: Separate the scramble into two halves. Garnish with fresh herbs if preferred and serve immediately.

Health Benefits:

➤ **Rich in Protein:** Eggs are a high-quality source of protein that promotes muscle repair and keeps you fuller for longer.
➤ **Packed with Vegetables**: The combination of bell peppers, spinach, zucchini, and mushrooms provides a variety of vitamins (A, C, K) and minerals such as potassium and magnesium.
➤ **High in Fiber:** The veggies in the scramble include fiber, which assists digestion and helps keep the gut healthy.
➤ **Low in Calories:** This meal contains relatively few calories, making it an excellent choice for weight control or loss.
➤ **Antioxidant:** Vegetables such as spinach and tomatoes are high in antioxidants, which help the immune system and fight free radicals.

Tips:

➤ **Egg Whites Option**: For a lighter version, substitute solely egg whites. This reduces fat and calories while maintaining a high protein level.
➤ **Extra Veggies:** Feel free to include any extra zero-point vegetables you choose, such as broccoli, kale, or asparagus.
➤ **Add a Spice Kick**: If you like spicy foods, add a sprinkle of chili flakes, paprika, or a splash of hot sauce for added flavor.
➤ **Meal Prep:** This scramble is ideal for meal preparation. You may chop all of your vegetables ahead of time and keep them in the refrigerator for convenient access throughout the week.
➤ **Cheese Option:** If you're not carefully tracking points or calories, add a little bit of low-fat cheese to the top before serving for extra richness.

Spinach and Mushroom Egg Muffins

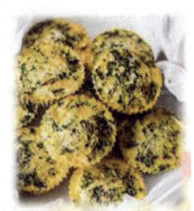

Prep Time: 10 minutes

Cooking Time: 15 minutes.

Total Time: 25 minutes.
Serving Size: 6 muffins

Ingredients:

- Six big eggs (or egg whites for a lower-calorie option)
- 1/2 cup chopped fresh spinach and 1/4 cup sliced mushrooms.
- 1/4 cup chopped onion.
- 1/4 cup chopped bell pepper.
- Season with salt and pepper to taste. - Add 1 tbsp olive oil or cooking spray (optional for sautéing).
- 1/4 teaspoon garlic powder (optional).

Directions:

1. Preheat the oven: Preheat the oven to 375°F (190°C). To prevent sticking, lightly grease a muffin pan with olive oil or spray with cooking spray.

2. Sauté mushrooms, onions, and bell pepper in olive oil or cooking spray for 3-4 minutes, until softened. Stir in the spinach and simmer for another 1–2 minutes, or until it is wilted. Remove from heat.

3. Prepare the eggs: Crack the eggs into a medium-sized bowl and whisk until thoroughly mixed. Season with salt, pepper, and garlic powder, if desired.

4. Incorporate Ingredients: Add sautéed veggies to the eggs and mix thoroughly to incorporate.

5. Fill the muffin pan equally with the egg and vegetable mixture, filling each cup approximately 3/4 full.

6. Bake: Place the muffin tray in the oven and bake for 15-18 minutes until the eggs are fully set and the tops are slightly brown.

7. Serve or Store: Allow the muffins to cool slightly before serving. You can also keep them in an airtight jar in the refrigerator for up to 4–5 days.

Health Benefits:

- **High in Protein:** Eggs are a high-quality source of protein that keeps you full and promotes muscular health.

- ➢ **High in Vegetables:** Spinach mushrooms and bell peppers include important vitamins and minerals such as vitamin K, vitamin C, and folate.
- ➢ **Low in Calories:** These muffins are ideal for individuals who want to maintain or reduce weight without losing taste or nutrients.
- ➢ **Portable:** Perfect for hectic mornings when you need a nutritious meal to go.

Tips:

- ➢ Add Cheese: For a creamier texture, put low-fat cheese on top of muffins before baking (may raise points).
- ➢ **Use silicone muffin cups:** They make clean-up easier and keep the muffins from sticking.
- ➢ **Batch Cooking:** These muffins freeze wonderfully, so make a big batch and freeze them for convenient breakfasts all week.

Overnight Chia Seed Pudding

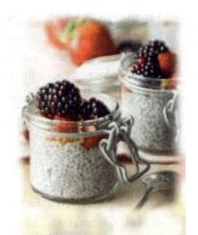

Prep Time: 5 minutes.
Cooking Time: None.

Total time is 5 minutes (plus 4-6 hours of chilling).
Servings: 2

Ingredients:

➢ 2 tablespoons chia seeds.
➢ One cup of unsweetened almond milk (or other plant-based milk)
➢ Add 1 tsp. vanilla essence and 1/2 tsp cinnamon (optional).
➢ 1 tablespoon maple syrup or your preferred sweetener (optional)
➢ Fresh fruit to top (berries, sliced banana, etc.)

Instructions:

1. Mix the Pudding
   In a small dish or container, mix together the chia seeds, almond milk, vanilla essence, cinnamon (if using), and maple syrup. Stir well to mix.

2. Refrigerate: Cover the bowl or jar and chill for at least 4 hours or overnight. During this time, the chia seeds will absorb the liquid, resulting in a thick, pudding-like texture.

3. Serve: When ready to serve, mix the pudding thoroughly. To enhance flavor and texture, top with fresh fruit like berries or sliced bananas.

Health benefits:

➢ Chia seeds have high levels of omega-3 fatty acids, which improve heart health and decrease inflammation.
➢ **Fiber-Rich:** Chia seeds are high in fiber, which aids digestion and keeps you feeling fuller for longer.
➢ **Bone Health:** Chia seeds are high in calcium; thus, this pudding is ideal for keeping healthy bones.
➢ **Antioxidants:** Chia seeds, cinnamon, and fresh fruit are high in antioxidants, which help protect your cells from harm.

Tips:

➢ **Customize the Sweetness:** Adjust the sweetness level by adding more or less maple syrup or your preferred sweetener.
➢ **Increase Protein:** Before serving, mix with a scoop of protein powder or Greek yogurt.
➢ **Make Ahead:** This pudding can be refrigerated for up to three days, making it an excellent meal prep choice.

Zucchini and Sweet Potato Hash

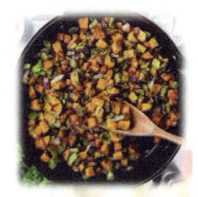

Prep Time: 10 minutes

Cooking Time: 15 minutes.

Total Time: 25 minutes.
Servings: 2

ingredients:

➤ Dice one medium zucchini and one medium sweet potato.
➤ Add 1/2 cup sliced onion, 1/2 cup diced bell pepper, and 1/4 tsp smoky paprika.
➤ 1/4 teaspoon garlic powder.
➤ Season with salt and pepper to taste. - Optional: 1 tablespoon olive oil or cooking spray.
➤ Fresh parsley as garnish (optional)

Directions:

1. Prepare Vegetables
  Peel and cut the sweet potato, zucchini, onion, and bell pepper into tiny, even pieces to ensure speedy and uniform cooking.

2. To cook the sweet potato, heat a large nonstick pan over medium heat. Add a splash of water or some olives oil/cooking spray. Add the sweet potato and cook for 6-7 minutes, stirring periodically, until it softens.

3. Add the remaining vegetables.
 Mix in the zucchini, onion, and bell pepper. Cook for 6-8 more minutes, stirring periodically, until all veggies are soft and gently browned.

4. Season with smoked paprika, garlic powder, salt, and pepper over the veggies. Stir well to get a uniform coating.

5. Serve: Divide the hash into two plates and sprinkle with fresh parsley as desired. Serve hot.

Health Benefits:

➤ **Rich in Vitamins:** Sweet potatoes include vitamin A, while zucchini and bell peppers contain vitamin C, which boosts immune function.
➤ **High in Fiber:** This meal aids digestion and creates a sense of fullness.
➤ **Low in Fat**: Made with little to no oil, this dish is both heart-healthy and low in calories.
➤ **Antioxidant Powerhouse:** The veggies in this hash are loaded with antioxidants, which fight inflammation and enhance overall wellness.

Tips:

Make it Spicy: Add a sprinkle of chili flakes or cayenne pepper for some spice.
Protein Boost: To boost protein, serve with a poached egg or lean turkey sausage.
Meal Prep: This hash keeps nicely in the fridge for up to three days. Simply reheat and enjoy.

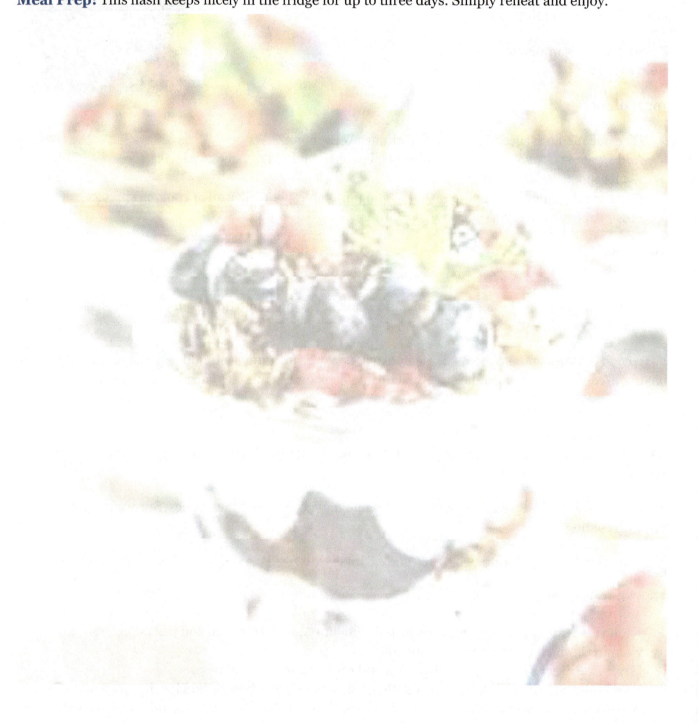

The Berry Blast Smoothie Bowl

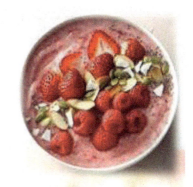

Prep Time: 5 minutes.
Cooking Time: None

Total Time: 5 min
Servings: 1

Ingredients:

> 1 cup frozen mixed berries (blueberries, raspberries, strawberries).
> 1/2 cup unsweetened almond milk (or other plant-based milk)
> One tiny sliced banana (optional for sweetness)
> 1/4 teaspoon vanilla extract.
> Fresh fruit to top (e.g., sliced kiwi, additional berries, banana)
> Optional toppings: chia seeds, shredded coconut, or slivered almonds (adjust points as needed).

Instructions:

1. Blend the Smoothie
   Blend together the frozen berries, almond milk, banana (if using), and vanilla essence. Blend until smooth and creamy. If necessary, add additional almond milk to get the desired consistency.

2. Assemble the Bowl: Pour the smoothie into a bowl and distribute evenly with a spoon.

3. Optional Toppings: Add fresh fruit, chia seeds, coconut, or almonds to the smoothie for extra texture and taste.

4. Serve: Eat immediately with a spoon.

Health Benefits:

> **Rich in Antioxidants:** Berries contain antioxidants that protect cells and improve skin health.
> **Low in Calories:** This dish is naturally low in calories yet high in nutrients.
> **Hydrating:** Berries and almond milk are high in water content, which helps you stay hydrated.
> **Helps with Digestion:** The fiber in the berries and banana aids digestive health.

Tips:

> **Freeze Your Banana:** To get a thicker, creamier consistency, freeze the banana.
> **Protein Boost:** To increase protein, add a scoop of protein powder to the blender.
> **Customizable Toppings:** Add granola, hemp seeds, or fresh mint leaves for a unique flavor.
> **Make ahead:** Make the smoothie blend the night before and keep it in the fridge. Simply add toppings in the morning.

CHAPTER TWO

FISH AND SEAFOOD

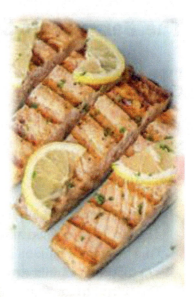

Lemon Garlic Grilled Salmon

Prep Time: 5 minutes.

Cooking Time: 10 minutes

Total Time: 15 minutes.
Servings: 2

ingredients:

- Two salmon fillets (4-6 ounces each, skin-on or skinless)
- 2 garlic cloves, minced
- 1 lemon, squeezed and zested
- 1 tbsp. fresh parsley, chopped (optional garnish)
- Add salt and pepper to taste.
- Olive oil spray or 1 tsp olive oil (optional; modify points as needed)

Directions:

1. Prepare marinade:
   In a small bowl, combine the garlic, lemon juice, zest, salt, and pepper. Set aside.

2. Marinate the salmon:
   Place the salmon fillets in a shallow dish or sealable bag. Pour the lemon-garlic mixture over the fillets, making sure it is evenly distributed. Allow the salmon to marinate for at least 10 minutes while you heat the grill.

3. Preheat the Grill: Set your grill or grill pan to medium-high heat. To avoid sticking, lightly coat the grill with olive oil spray.

4. Grill the Salmon: Place salmon fillets on the grill, skin-side down (if applicable). Cook for 4-5 minutes per side, or until the salmon flakes easily with a fork and is well charred. Avoid overcooking the fish to keep it moist.

5. Serve the cooked salmon on a dish with garnishes. Garnish with fresh parsley and a lemon wedge if preferred. Serve immediately.

Health Benefits:

➢ **Rich in Omega-3 Fatty Acids**: Salmon contains heart-healthy omega-3s that lower inflammation and improve cognitive health.
➢ **High in Protein:** An excellent protein source to keep you full and boost muscular health.
➢ **Low in Calories:** Grilling keeps the meal light and nutritious.
➢ **Vitamin Boost:** Lemon juice gives vitamin C, while salmon contains critical B vitamins.

Tips:

➢ **Use a Grill Pan:** If you don't have an outside grill, a stovetop grill pan is ideal.
➢ **Make it spicy:** For a spicy marinade, add a sprinkle of chili flakes or cayenne pepper.
➢ **Pair It:** To complete the meal, serve the salmon with steamed vegetables, cauliflower rice, or a fresh salad.
➢ **Check for Doneness:** Salmon is done when the interior temperature reaches 145°F (63°C).

Lemon Garlic Grilled Salmon is a simple, healthful, and tasty recipe that is ideal for lunch or dinner. This dinner is a great addition to the Zero Point Lifestyle and can be enjoyed by the entire family.

Shrimp and Avocado Lettuce Wraps

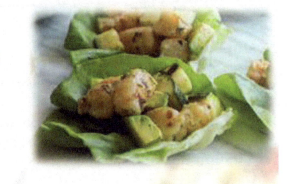

Preparation Time: 10 minutes

Cooking Time: 5 min
Total Time: fifteen minutes
Servings: 2

Ingredients:

- 1/2 lb. (225 g) peeled and deveined big shrimp, 1/2 tsp smoked paprika.
- 1/4 teaspoon garlic powder.
- Add salt and pepper to taste.
- Olive oil spray or 1 teaspoon olive oil (optional)
- One avocado, diced
- One tablespoon lime juice.
- 6 big lettuce leaves (such as romaine, butter, or iceberg)
- Fresh cilantro or parsley as a garnish.

Directions:

1. Prepare Shrimp: Sprinkle the shrimp with smoked paprika, garlic powder, salt, and pepper.

2. Cook the Shrimp: Heat a non-stick pan over medium heat and generously coat with olive oil (or use 1 tsp.). Cook the shrimp for 2–3 minutes per side until pink and cooked through. Remove from heat.

3. Prepare Avocado: In a small bowl, combine the chopped avocado, lime juice, salt, and pepper to taste.

4. Assemble the wraps by laying the lettuce leaves flat and equally dividing the cooked shrimp and diced avocado among them.

5. Garnish with fresh cilantro or parsley and serve immediately.

Health Benefits:

- **Low-Calorie Protein**: Shrimp is a lean, protein-rich food with low calories.
- **Heart-Healthy Fats:** Avocado contains monounsaturated fats, which promote heart health.
- **Vitamin Boost:** Lettuce and lime juice provide vitamins A, C, and K.
- **Gluten-Free and Keto-Friendly:** An adaptable recipe for a variety of dietary requirements.

Tips:

- **Make It Spicy:** Add spicy sauce or chili flakes for more spice.
- **Add Crunch:** For texture, mix with thinly sliced radishes or shredded carrots.

Baked Cod with Herb Crust

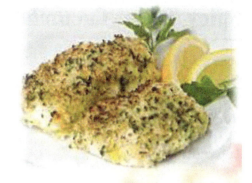

Prep Time: 10 minutes

Cooking Time: 20 minutes

Total Time: 30 minutes.
Servings: 2

Ingredients:

➢ Two cod fillets (4-6 ounces each)
➢ To prepare, carefully cut 1/4 cup fresh parsley, 1/4 cup fresh dill, and mince 1 clove garlic.
➢ Add 1 tbsp. lemon zest and 1 tbsp. Dijon mustard.
➢ 1/4 teaspoon salt.
➢ 1/4 teaspoon black pepper.
➢ Olive oil spray or 1 teaspoon olive oil (optional)

Directions:

1. Preheat the oven. Preheat the oven to 400°F (200°C). Cover a baking sheet with parchment paper or gently oil it.

2. Prepare Herb Mixture: In a small bowl, mix together parsley, dill, garlic, lemon zest, Dijon mustard, salt, and pepper.

3. Coat the fish fillets: Place the fish fillets on the prepared baking sheet. Evenly distribute the herb mixture on top of each fillet.

4. Bake the fish: Bake in a preheated oven for 18-20 minutes, or until the fish flakes easily with a fork and is fully done.

5. To serve, place the fish on a dish and decorate with lemon wedges or fresh herbs. Serve hot.

Health Benefits:

➢ **Rich in Protein**: Cod is a lean source of high-quality protein, which promotes muscular health.
➢ **Low in Calories:** Ideal for weight control and a healthy diet.
➢ **Packed with Nutrients:** Fresh herbs and fish include critical vitamins and minerals, including B12, selenium, and potassium.
➢ **Heart-Healthy:** Cod is low in fat, making it an excellent option for cardiovascular health.

Tips:

➢ **Use Other Herbs:** Replace parsley and dill with basil, thyme, or chives for a unique taste profile.
➢ **Pair it**: To finish the dish, serve with steamed veggies, a side salad, or roasted sweet potatoes.
➢ **Check for Completeness:** Cod is ready when the interior temperature reaches 145°F (63°C).

Spicy Tuna, Cucumber Bites

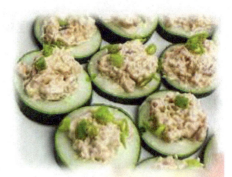

Prep Time: 10 minutes.
Cooking time: None
Total Time: 10 minutes
Servings: 4 (makes approximately 16 bites).

Ingredients:

- 1 can (5 oz) tuna in water, drained
- 2 tablespoons nonfat plain Greek yogurt
- 1 tsp. sriracha or spicy sauce (to taste)
- 1/4 teaspoon garlic powder.
- 1/4 teaspoon smoked paprika.
- One cucumber, cut into rounds (approximately 16 slices)
- Season to taste with salt and pepper.
- Optional garnishes include chopped green onion or sesame seeds.

Directions:

1. Prepare Tuna Mixture: In a medium mixing bowl, add drained tuna, Greek yogurt, sriracha, garlic powder, smoked paprika, salt, and pepper. Mix well until creamy and evenly blended.

2. Cucumber Slice: Cut the cucumber into 1/4 inch thick rounds and place on a serving plate.

3. Assemble the Bites: Add a tiny quantity of tuna mixture to each cucumber slice.

4. Garnish and Serve: Top each bite with chopped green onion or sesame seeds for added flavor and appearance. Serve immediately.

Health Benefits:

- **Low Calories:** Cucumber and tuna are low-calorie, nutrient-dense meals.
- **Protein-Packed:** Tuna has a lot of lean protein, which helps you stay full for longer.
- **High in Omega-3s:** Tuna contains vital omega-3 fatty acids, which promote heart and brain function.
- **Hydrating:** Cucumbers have a high water content, which promotes hydration.

Tips:

- **Add a Crunch:** Top with a tiny slice of red bell pepper or radish for added texture.
- **Spice Levels:** Adjust the quantity of sriracha to your liking.
- **Meal Prep:** Prepare the tuna mixture ahead of time, and then assemble the bites right before serving.

Coconut Lime Shrimp Soup

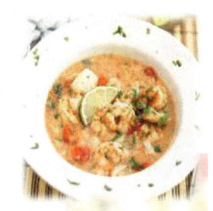

Prep Time: 10 minutes

Cooking Time: 15 minutes

Total Time: 25 minutes.
Servings: 4

Ingredients:

➢ 1/2 lb (225 g) peeled and deveined giant shrimp, 1 can (14 oz) light coconut milk.
➢ To prepare, combine 2 cups of low-sodium chicken or veggie broth, 1 tbsp grated fresh ginger, and 2 minced garlic cloves.
➢ Two tablespoons of fresh lime juice
➢ 1 tablespoon of fish sauce (optional for depth of flavor)
➢ 1/2 tsp red chili flakes (adjust for taste)
➢ 1 cup sliced mushrooms.
➢ 1/2 cup cherry tomatoes (halved)
➢ 1/4 cup fresh cilantro, chopped (plus more for garnish)
➢ Add salt and pepper to taste.

Directions:

1. Sauté Aromatics: In a large saucepan over medium heat, sauté the garlic and ginger with a splash of broth until fragrant, about 1 minute.

2. Combine Broth and Coconut Milk: Add the chicken or veggie broth and coconut milk. Bring to a moderate simmer.

3. Cook the Vegetables: Place the mushrooms and cherry tomatoes in the saucepan. Simmer for 5 minutes, until the veggies are soft.

4. Add Shrimp: Combine shrimp, lime juice, fish sauce (optional), chili flakes, salt, and pepper. Cook for 3-4 minutes, or until the shrimp are pink and cooked through.

5. Finish with Cilantro: Add chopped cilantro and adjust spice as required.

6. Serve: Ladle soup into dishes and top with more cilantro. Serve hot.

Health Benefits:

➢ Rich in Protein: Shrimp contains lean protein that aids in muscle growth and repair.
➢ Low in Fat: Using light coconut milk maintains the meal's creaminess while reducing saturated fats.
➢ Boosts Immunity: Ginger, garlic, and lime juice include antioxidants that stimulate the immune system.

➤ Hydrating and Nourishing: The broth is hydrating and nutrient-rich.

Tips:

➤ Add Veggies: Add spinach, zucchini, or bok choy for extra nutrition and bulk.
➤ Spice It Up: Increase the spiciness by adjusting the chili flakes or adding a dash of chile oil.
➤ Storage: This soup keeps nicely in the refrigerator for up to three days. Reheat slightly before serving.

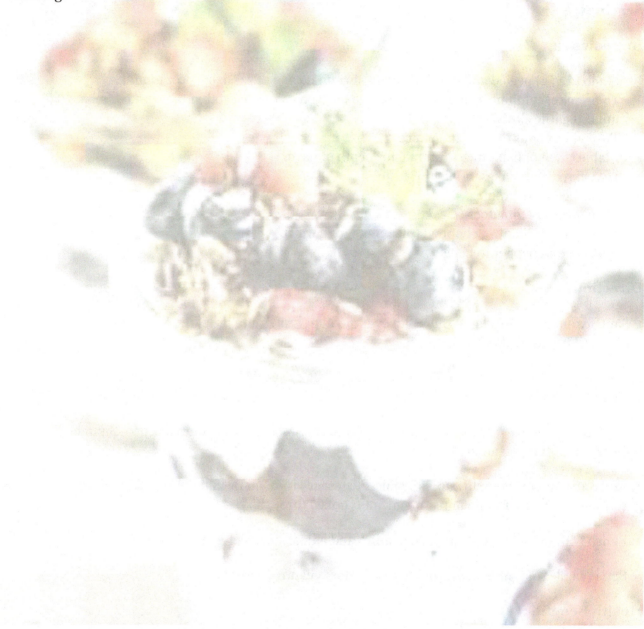

CHAPTER THREE

BEEF

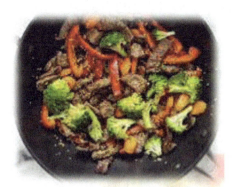

Zero-Point Beef and Vegetable Stir-Fry

Prep Time: 10 minutes

Cooking Time: 10 minutes

Total Time: 20 minutes.
Servings: 4

ingredients:

- 1 lb (450 g) of lean beef strips (sirloin, flank, or tenderloin) and 2 cups of broccoli florets.
- 1 thinly sliced red bell pepper, 1 cup snap peas, 1 julienned medium carrot, 1 thinly sliced small onion, and 2 minced garlic cloves.
- 1 tsp fresh ginger, grated
- Three tablespoons of low-sodium soy sauce.
- 2 tbsp rice vinegar, 1 tbsp oyster sauce (optional for flavor depth).
- 1/2 teaspoon of red pepper flakes (optional for spice)
- Olive oil spray or 1 teaspoon olive oil (optional)
- Fresh cilantro or green onions as garnish

Directions:

1. Prepare the meat: - Cut meat into thin strips if not pre-cut. Season gently with salt and pepper.

2. Cook the Beef: Preheat a large nonstick skillet or wok to high heat. Spray gently with olive oil or use 1 tsp.
Cook the beef strips for 2-3 minutes, tossing regularly, until browned. Remove from the skillet and put aside.

3. Sauté vegetables: Cook garlic and ginger in the same pan for 30 seconds until aromatic.
Combine the broccoli, bell pepper, snap peas, carrots, and onion. Stir-fry for 3-5 minutes, until the veggies are soft and crisp.

4. Make the Sauce: - In a small mixing bowl, combine the soy sauce, rice vinegar, and oyster sauce (if using).

5. Combine and Cook: Return the steak to the skillet and pour the sauce over it.
If you like it hot, add red pepper flakes. Stir well and cook for another 2 minutes, until everything is coated and cooked thoroughly.

6. Garnish and Serve: Remove from heat, garnish with fresh cilantro or green onions, and serve right away.

Health Benefits:

> **Lean Protein:** Beef is high in protein, which promotes muscle regeneration and general health.
> **Nutrient-Dense Veggies:** Broccoli, carrots, and bell peppers include fiber, vitamins, and antioxidants.
> **Low in Calories:** A balanced, full meal that aids with weight management.
> **Heart-Healthy:** Low in bad fats, particularly when using lean meat.

Tips: -

> Customize Your Vegetables for added variety, use zucchini, mushrooms, or asparagus.
> **Prepare ahead:** To speed up the cooking process, chop veggies and slice meat beforehand.
> **Service Options:** Enjoy as is, or with cauliflower rice or lettuce wraps for a zero-point meal.
> **Storage:** Keep leftovers in an airtight jar for up to three days. Reheat in a skillet for the best results.

Classic Beef and Tomato Stew

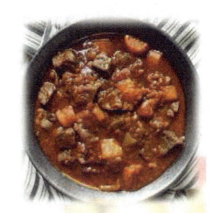

Prep Time: 15 minutes

Cooking Time: 1 hour 30 minutes

Total Time: 1 hour and 45 minutes.
Servings: 4

Ingredients:

➤ 1 pound (450 grams) of lean beef stew meat, trimmed of fat
➤ one medium onion, diced
➤ 2 garlic cloves, minced
➤ one big carrot, chopped
➤ Two celery stalks, chopped
➤ 1 cup chopped tomatoes, either canned or fresh.
➤ 2 cups low-sodium beef broth and 1 tablespoon tomato paste.
➤ 1 teaspoon paprika.
➤ Add 1 tsp dried thyme and 1 bay leaf.
➤ Add salt and pepper to taste.
➤ 1/4 cup freshly chopped parsley (for garnish)

Directions:

1. Sear the Beef
   preheat a big saucepan or Dutch oven to medium-high heat. Use a thin spray of olive oil (optional).
   Cook the meat until it is browned on both sides, about 5 minutes. Remove and set aside.

2. Sauté vegetables in the same saucepan. Add onion, garlic, carrot, and celery. Cook for 3-5 minutes, until softened.

3. Build the Stew: - Combine chopped tomatoes, tomato paste, paprika, thyme, bay leaf, and beef broth. Stir thoroughly.
   Return the meat to the pot.

4. Simmer: Bring mixture to a boil, then lower to a low simmer. Cover and simmer for 1.5 hours, stirring regularly, until the meat is cooked and the flavors have combined.

5. Season and Serve: Remove the bay leaf, season with salt and pepper, and garnish with fresh parsley before serving.

Health Benefits:

➤ **High in Protein:** Beef contains important amino acids for muscular development and repair.

- ➢ **Nutrient-Rich Vegetables:** Carrots, celery, and tomatoes provide vitamins, fiber, and antioxidants.
- ➢ **Low-Calorie:** A filling dinner without excessive calories.

Tips:

- ➢ **Increase Veggies:** Add potatoes, green beans, or zucchini for variation.
- ➢ **Storage:** It keeps nicely in the refrigerator for up to three days. Freezes effectively for up to three months.
- ➢ **Service Suggestion:** Enjoy alone or with cauliflower rice for a zero-point supper.

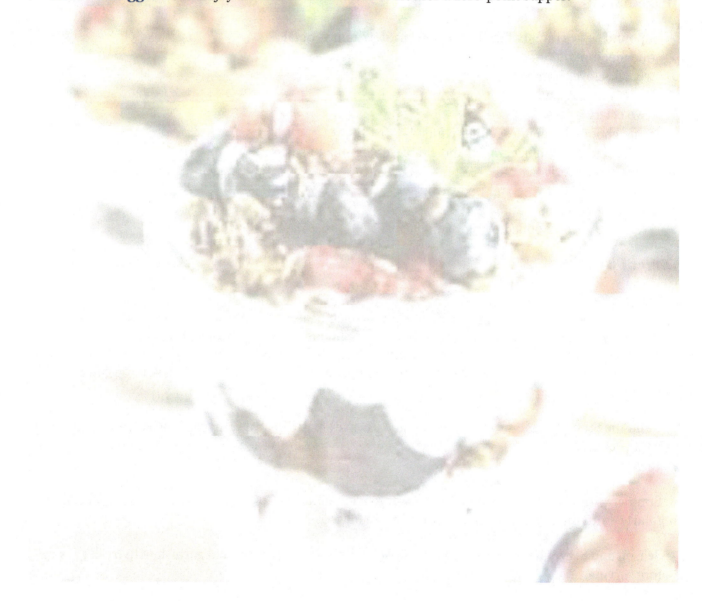

Spicy Beef Lettuce Wraps

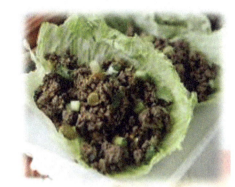

Prep Time: 10 minutes.
Cook Time: 10 minutes
Total Time: 20 minutes
Servings: 4 (creates 8 wraps)

Ingredients:

- 1 lb. (450 g) lean ground beef, 1 finely diced onion, and 2 minced garlic cloves.
- 1 teaspoon ground cumin.
- 1/2 teaspoon smoked paprika.
- 1/2 teaspoon chili powder.
- 1/4 teaspoon of cayenne pepper (optional for heat)
- 1/4 cup fresh cilantro, chopped
- 8 big lettuce leaves (butter lettuce or romaine are ideal)
- Optional toppings include chopped tomatoes, sliced radishes, shredded carrots, and lime wedges.

Directions:

1. Cook the Beef: Cook in a nonstick skillet over medium heat. Combine the ground meat and onion. Cook for approximately 5-7 minutes, or until the steak has browned and the onion has softened.

2. Season the meat with garlic, cumin, smoked paprika, chili powder, and cayenne pepper (optional). Stir thoroughly and simmer for another 2 minutes.
Remove from the fire and stir in the chopped cilantro.

3. Assemble the Wraps: Spoon the seasoned beef mixture onto the lettuce leaves.
 If wanted, top with your favorite toppings.

4. Serve: Arrange on a dish and serve immediately with lime wedges for added flavor.

Health Benefits:

- **High Protein:** Ground beef is an excellent source of lean protein.
- **Low-Carb:** Using lettuce leaves rather than bread or tortillas reduces carbohydrates.
- **Nutrient Boost:** Toppings such as radishes and tomatoes provide vitamins and antioxidants.

Tips: -

- **Meal Prep**: Prepare the beef mixture ahead of time and reheat before constructing wraps.
- **Make It Spicy:** To increase the spiciness, add sliced jalapeños or cayenne pepper.
- **Serve with dip:** For an extra taste boost, serve with a zero-point yogurt sauce.

Both dishes are easy to create, full of flavor, and perfect for a zero-point lifestyle!

Grilled beef with chimichurri sauce

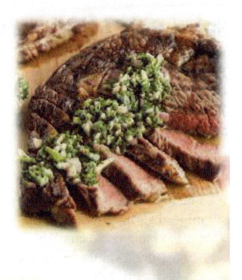

Prep Time: 15 minutes

Cooking Time: 10 minutes

Total Time: 25 minutes.
Servings: 4

Ingredients:

For Beef:

➤ 1 pound (450 grams) lean beef steaks (sirloin or flank)
➤ Add salt and pepper to taste.

For Chimichurri Sauce:

➤ To prepare, carefully cut 1/2 cup fresh parsley, 1/4 cup fresh cilantro, and mince 3 garlic cloves.
➤ Two tablespoons of red wine vinegar.
➤ 1/4 teaspoon red pepper flakes.
➤ Juice from 1 lime
➤ Add salt and pepper to taste.

Directions:

1. To make the chimichurri sauce, combine parsley, cilantro, garlic, red wine vinegar, lime juice, and red pepper flakes. Season with salt and pepper to taste. Allow the sauce to sit for 10 minutes so that the flavors may combine.

2. Season the meat: - Pat dries the meat and seasons both sides with salt and pepper.

3. Grill the Beef: Preheat a grill or grill pan on high heat.
Grill the steaks for 3-5 minutes on each side, or until desired doneness.
Take the steaks from the grill and allow them to rest for 5 minutes before slicing.

4. To serve, slice the beef against the grain and sprinkle with chimichurri sauce.

Health Benefits:

➤ **Lean Protein:** Beef contains key elements such as iron and zinc.
➤ **Antioxidant-Rich Sauce:** Chimichurri sauce contains herbs and garlic that have anti-inflammatory qualities.
➤ **Low-Calorie and Nutrient-Dense:** A healthy option for weight management and general well-being.

Tips:

➢ **Marinade Bonus:** Use some of the chimichurri sauce to marinate the meat before grilling.
➢ **Make ahead:** For a more intense taste, prepare the sauce up to 24 hours ahead of time.
➢ **Serving Ideas:** Serve with roasted veggies or a simple green salad.

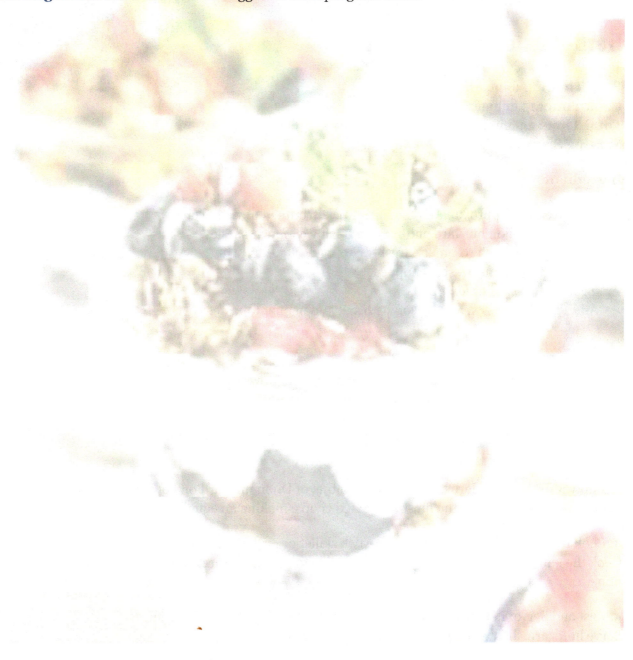

CHAPTER FOUR

PORK AND LAMB

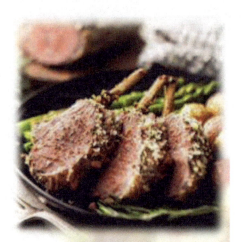

Herb-crusted lamb chops

Prep Time: 10 minutes.
Cook Time: 15 minutes
Total Time: 25 minutes
Serving Size: 4 (2 chops per serving)

Ingredients:

- 8 lamb chops (approximately one inch thick, trimmed of visible fat)
- Add 2 tbsp. Dijon mustard and 1/2 cup freshly chopped parsley.
- 2 tablespoons fresh rosemary, freshly chopped
- 2 tbsp. fresh thyme, freshly chopped
- 2 garlic cloves, minced
- Add 1 tsp. lemon zest and season with salt and pepper to taste.

Directions:

1. Prepare lamb chops by patting them dry with a paper towel.
 Season each side gently with salt and pepper.

2. Prepare the herb coating: In a small bowl, combine the parsley, rosemary, thyme, garlic, and lemon zest.

3. Apply Mustard and Herbs: Apply a thin coating of Dijon mustard on both sides of the lamb chops.
Apply the herb mixture to the mustard-coated chops, making an equal coating.

4. Cook the Lamb Chops: Preheat a non-stick skillet or grill pan to medium-high heat.
Cook the lamb chops for 3-4 minutes on each side for medium-rare, or longer if you want them well-done.

5. Rest and Serve: Let the lamb chops rest for 5 minutes to disperse their juices.
Serve hot, garnished with more fresh herbs as desired.

Health Benefits:

- **Lean Protein**: Lamb provides high-quality protein.

- ➤ **Rich in Vitamins and Minerals:** Lamb contains B vitamins, zinc, and iron, which are necessary for energy and immunological health.
- ➤ **Herb Power:** Fresh herbs such as parsley, rosemary, and thyme have antioxidants and anti-inflammatory effects.

Tips:

- ➤ **Temperature Check:** Use a meat thermometer for precise results: 145°F (63°C) for medium-rare and 160°F (71°C) for medium.
- ➤ **Pairing Suggestions:** Pair with roasted veggies or a fresh green salad for a zero-point supper.
- ➤ **Advance Preparation:** Coat the lamb chops with mustard and herbs up to 4 hours ahead of time and store until ready to cook.

These lamb chops are fast, tasty, and suitable for both regular dinners and special occasions!

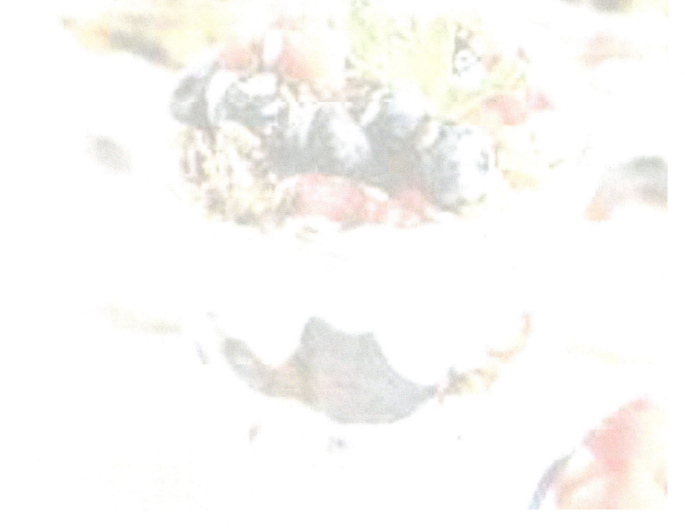

Pork Tenderloin with Apple Slaw

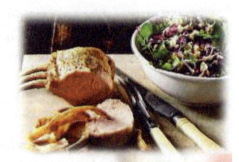

Prep Time: 15 minutes

Cooking Time: 25 minutes

Total Time: 40 minutes.
Servings: 4

Ingredients:

For Pork Tenderloin:

➤ 1 pound (450 grams) pork tenderloin, trimmed of visible fat
➤ 2 tsp olive oil (optional, to coat pan)
➤ One teaspoon of smoked paprika.
➤ One teaspoon of garlic powder.
➤ 1/2 teaspoon ground cumin.
➤ Add salt and pepper to taste.

For Apple Slaw:

➤ 2 medium apples, julienned (Granny Smith or Honeycrisp are ideal)
➤ 1/2 finely shredded small red cabbage, 1 grated medium carrot, and 2 tablespoons apple cider vinegar.
➤ 1 tbsp Dijon mustard, 1 tbsp fresh lemon juice.
➤ Add salt and pepper to taste.

Directions:

For Pork Tenderloin:
1. Preheat Oven: Preheat the oven to 400°F (200°C).
2. Season the Pork: In a small bowl, combine the paprika, garlic powder, cumin, salt, and pepper. Rub the spice evenly over the pork tenderloin.
3. Sear the Pork: Preheat a large pan to medium-high heat. If required, sprinkle with olive oil and sear the pork on all sides until browned (approximately 2-3 minutes per side).
4. Roast the Pork: Place the pork on a baking dish and bake for 20-25 minutes, or until the internal temperature reaches 145°F (63°C).
5. Rest and Slice: Allow the pork to rest for 5 minutes before slicing into medallions.

For Apple Slaw:
1. Prepare Slaw: In a large bowl, mix the julienned apples, shredded cabbage, and grated carrot.
2. Prepare the dressing: In a small bowl, combine the apple cider vinegar, Dijon mustard, lemon juice, salt, and pepper.
3. Toss together. Pour the dressing over the apple slaw and toss to evenly coat.

Serve the pork medallions with a big serving of apple slaw.

Health Benefits:

- ➤ **Lean Protein:** Pork tenderloin is a low-fat and protein-rich option.
- ➤ **High in Fiber:** The apple slaw provides fiber as well as a nutritional boost.
- ➤ **Immune Support:** Apples and cabbage contain antioxidants, which promote general health.

Tips:

- ➤ **Make Ahead:** For a more flavorful apple slaw, make it a few hours ahead.
- ➤ **Serving Suggestion:** Serve with roasted sweet potatoes for a more substantial dinner.
- ➤ **Leftovers:** Pack leftover pork and slaw into lettuce wraps for a fast lunch!

Spicy Lamb Meatballs with Tomato Sauce

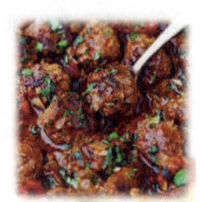

Prep Time: 15 minutes.
Cook Time: 30 minutes
Total Time: 45 minutes
Serve Size: 4 (4-5 meatballs per serve)

Ingredients:

For the meatballs:

➤ One pound (450 grams) of lean ground lamb
➤ 1/4 cup coarsely grated onion and 2 chopped garlic cloves.
➤ 1 tsp. ground cumin, 1 tsp. smoked paprika.
➤ 1/2 teaspoon ground coriander.
➤ 1/4 tsp. cayenne pepper (optional for additional heat)
➤ Chop 1 tbsp. fresh parsley. - Season with salt and pepper to taste.

For Tomato Sauce:

➤ To prepare, combine 1 can (14 oz./400 g) crushed tomatoes, 1/2 cup finely chopped onion, and 2 minced garlic cloves.
➤ 1 teaspoon of olive oil (optional for sautéing)
➤ One teaspoon dried oregano.
➤ 1/2 teaspoon of crushed red pepper flakes (optional)
➤ Add salt and pepper to taste.

Directions:

For the meatballs:
1. Combine the meatball ingredients: In a large mixing bowl, add the ground lamb, shredded onion, garlic, cumin, smoked paprika, coriander, cayenne pepper, parsley, salt, and pepper. Mix until just mixed.
2. Form Meatballs: Roll the mixture into tiny balls (approximately an inch in diameter). You should have 16 to 20 meatballs.

Sauce Directions:

3. Sauté Aromatics: Heat a skillet on medium heat. Sauté the onion and garlic until aromatic (approximately 3-4 minutes), then add the olive oil.
4. Simmering the Sauce: Combine the crushed tomatoes, oregano, red pepper flakes, salt, and pepper. Stir and boil for 10 minutes.

Cook the meatballs:
5. Add to Sauce: Carefully drop the meatballs in the tomato sauce.

6. Simmer: Cover and cook the meatballs for 15-20 minutes, turning them regularly to ensure they cook evenly.

Serving Instructions: Serve the meatballs and sauce hot, topped with more parsley if preferred.

Health Benefits:

➢ **Rich in Protein**: Lamb contains high-quality protein and vital minerals such as iron and zinc.
➢ **Low in Added Fat:** The meatballs are lean and prepared in a light tomato sauce.
➢ **Heart-Healthy Tomatoes:** Tomatoes contain several antioxidants, including lycopene.

Tip:

➢ **Make Ahead:** Freeze meatballs and sauce for up to three months.
➢ **Serving Ideas:** Serve with zucchini noodles or steamed veggies for a full dinner.
➢ **Adjust Spice:** For a milder taste, omit the cayenne and red pepper flakes.

Both dishes are nutritious, tasty, and suitable for a zero-point diet!

Zero Point Pulled Pork Lettuce Wraps

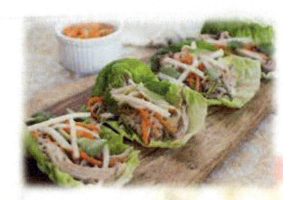

Preparation Time: 10 minutes

Cooking Time: 6–8 hours (slow cooker) or 1 hour (pressure cooker).
Total time: varies depending on the cooking technique.
Serving Size: 6 (2 wraps per serving)

ingredients:

For the Pulled Pork:

- 2 pounds (900 grams) of pork shoulder, trimmed of visible fat.
- One medium onion, cut
- 3 garlic cloves, minced
- 1 cup of chicken broth (low sodium)
- 1/4 cup apple cider vinegar.
- One tablespoon of smoked paprika.
- 1 tsp. ground cumin, 1 tsp. chili powder.
- 1/2 teaspoon ground black pepper.
- Salt to taste.

For the wraps:

- Large lettuce leaves (butter lettuce or romaine are excellent).
- 1/2 cup grated carrots (optional)
- 1/2 cup sliced red bell pepper (optional).
- Fresh cilantro for garnish.
- Lime wedges for serving.

Directions:

For the Pulled Pork:
1. Prepare Pork: Season the pork shoulder with smoked paprika, cumin, chili powder, black pepper, and salt.
2. Slow Cooker Method: Place onion slices and minced garlic in the bottom of the slow cooker.
Place the seasoned pork shoulder on top. Add the chicken broth and apple cider vinegar.
Cover and simmer on low for 6-8 hours, or until the pork is soft enough to shred with a fork.
3. Pressure Cooker Method: Brown the pork on both sides using the sauté function. Remove and set aside.
To deglaze the saucepan, add the onion, garlic, stock, and vinegar. Return the meat, shut the lid, and cook for 1 hour under high pressure. Use a natural pressure release.

4. Shred the meat: Remove the meat and shred using two forks. Return the shredded pork to the cooking liquids for more flavors.

Step 5: Assemble the wraps. Spoon the pulled pork onto lettuce leaves. Garnish with shredded carrots, diced bell peppers, and fresh cilantro.
6. Service: Serve with lime wedges for a refreshing, acidic kick.

Health Benefits:

➢ **Lean Protein:** Trimming fat from pork shoulder results in a tasty and protein-rich choice.
➢ **Low-Carb:** Lettuce wraps substitute typical tortillas for a lighter, lower-carb option.
➢ **Nutritional Boost:** Fresh vegetables provide vitamins and antioxidants.

Tips:

➢ **Make It Ahead:** Prepare pulled pork ahead of time and refrigerate for up to three days.
➢ **Spice It Up:** Add a dab of spicy sauce or chili flakes for an added kick.
➢ **Alternative Toppings:** For a tangier flavor, try pickled onions or a dollop of Greek yogurt.

Garlic and herb pork medallions

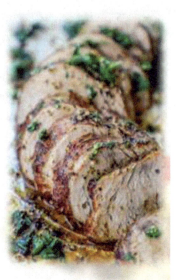

Prep Time: 10 minutes

Cooking Time: 15 minutes

Total Time: 25 minutes.
Servings: 4

ingredients:

➢ 1 pound (450 grams) pork tenderloin, cut into 1-inch-thick medallions.
➢ 2 garlic cloves, minced
➢ 1 tablespoon fresh rosemary, freshly chopped
➢ 1 tbsp fresh thyme, freshly chopped
➢ To prepare, add 1/2 tsp lemon zest, salt and pepper to taste, and 1 tsp olive oil (optional for cooking).

Directions:

1. Prepare the Pork Medallions: - Season the pork medallions with salt, pepper, rosemary, thyme, garlic, and lemon zest.

2. To cook the medallions, prepare a nonstick pan over medium-high heat. Add a tiny bit of olive oil if necessary.
Sear the pork medallions for 2-3 minutes per side, or until browned and internal temperature reaches 145°F (63°C).

3. Rest and Serve: Remove medallions from pan and allow to rest for 5 minutes before serving.

Health Benefits: -

➢ **Lean Protein:** Pork tenderloin has minimal fat and high protein content.
➢ **Heart-Healthy Herbs:** Rosemary and thyme are high in antioxidants and anti-inflammatory properties.
➢ **Quick Cooking:** Because of the short cooking time, this food keeps nutrients well.

Tips:

➢ **Side Pairings:** Pair with steamed asparagus or roasted sweet potatoes for a complete dinner.
➢ **Make It Zesty:** To add brightness, squeeze fresh lemon juice over the medallions before serving.
➢ **Meal Prep:** These medallions reheat nicely and make great leftovers for salads and wraps.

Both recipes are easy, healthy, and full of taste, helping you maintain your zero-point lifestyle!

CHAPTER FIVE

POULTRY

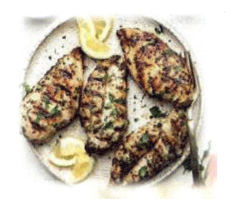

Lemon Herb Grilled Chicken Breast

Preparation Time: 10 minutes

Marinating Time: 30 minutes (optional but encouraged)
Cook Time: 8-10 minutes
Duration: 20-40 minutes
Servings: 4

Ingredients:

- 4 boneless, skinless chicken breasts (about 6 oz each)
- Two tablespoons of olive oil.
- Juice and zest of one lemon
- 2 garlic cloves, minced
- 1 tbsp fresh thyme, freshly chopped
- 1 tablespoon fresh rosemary, freshly chopped
- One teaspoon dried oregano.
- Add salt and pepper to taste.

Directions:

1. Marinate chicken with olive oil, lemon juice and zest, garlic, thyme, rosemary, oregano, salt, and pepper.
Place the chicken breasts in a shallow dish or resalable bag, and then pour the marinade over them.
Toss to coat evenly.
Allow the chicken to marinate for at least 30 minutes (up to 4 hours in the fridge for more flavor).

2. Preheat the Grill: - Set your grill or grill pan to medium-high heat.
If using an outside grill, grease the grates to keep them from sticking.

3. Grill the Chicken: - Take the chicken out of the marinade and discard it.
Grill the chicken breasts for 4-5 minutes on each side, or until the internal temperature reaches 165°F (74°C).
The chicken can also be cooked on a stovetop grill pan.

4. Rest and Serve: After cooking, let the chicken rest for 5 minutes before slicing.
  - Serve hot alongside grilled veggies or a fresh salad.

Health Benefits:

➢ **Lean Protein**: Low-fat, high-protein chicken breast promotes muscle growth and repair.
➢ **Heart-Healthy Herbs**: Rosemary, thyme, and oregano have anti-inflammatory compounds that may aid digestion.
➢ **Low in Calories:** With little additional fat, this meal is light but rich in taste.

Tips:

➢ **Marinating Time:** To enhance taste, marinate chicken for 2-4 hours. If you're in a hurry, 30 minutes still delivers amazing flavor!
➢ **Grill markings:** To get excellent grill markings; avoid moving the chicken around on the grill too frequently.
➢ **Serve with Sides:** For a complete supper, serve this grilled chicken with quinoa salad or roasted veggies.
➢ **Make it spicy:** To add some spice, add a sprinkle of red pepper flakes or cayenne pepper to the marinade.

This Lemon Herb Grilled Chicken Breast dish is easy, full of fresh tastes, and a fantastic way to keep to your zero-point diet while still having a fulfilling dinner!

Turkey and Zucchini Meatballs

Prep Time: 15 minutes.
Cook Time: 25 minutes.
Total Time: forty minutes
Serving Size: 4 (12 meatballs)
Points per Recipe: 0 (0 points)

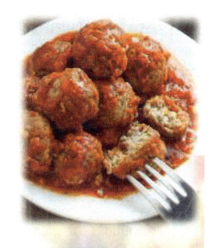

Ingredients:

- 1 lb (450 g) lean ground turkey
- 1 cup shredded zucchini (squeeze to remove extra moisture)
- one egg, beaten
- 1/4 cup finely chopped onion.
- 2 garlic cloves, minced
- 1/4 cup fresh parsley, chopped
- 1/2 teaspoon dried oregano.
- 1/2 tsp salt and 1/4 tsp black pepper.

Directions:

1. Preheat the oven to 400°F (200°C). Line a baking sheet with parchment paper or gently coat with cooking oil.

2. Mix the meatballs. In a large mixing bowl, add ground turkey, grated zucchini, egg, onion, garlic, parsley, oregano, salt, and pepper. Mix well until all components are uniformly distributed.

3. Form the Meatballs: - Using your hands or a small scoop, shape the mixture into 12 evenly-sized balls. Place them on the prepared baking sheet.

4. Bake the Meatballs: - Bake in a preheated oven for 20-25 minutes, or until the internal temperature reaches 165°F (74°C).

5. Serve: Serve the meatballs with marinara sauce, zucchini noodles, or a fresh salad.

Health Benefits:

- **Lean Protein:** Turkey's high protein and low fat content promote muscular health.
- **Hydrating Vegetable:** Zucchini provides hydration and nutrients without adding calories.
- **Gluten-Free:** Naturally gluten-free and ideal for a clean eating regimen.

Tips:

- **Make It Spicy:** Add red pepper flakes for a touch of spiciness.
- **Meal Preparation:** These meatballs store nicely for up to three months. Just reheat as required.
- **Service Options:** For a delicious dip, serve with tzatziki or salsa made with yogurt.

Balsamic Glazed Chicken Thighs

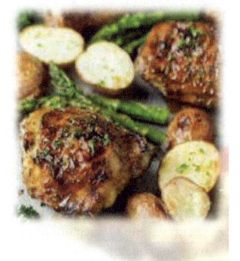

Prep Time: 10 minutes

Cooking Time: 25 minutes

Total Time: 35 minutes.
Servings: 4

Ingredients:

- 1 1/2 pounds (700 grams) of boneless, skinless chicken thighs.
- 1/4 cup balsamic vinegar.
- 2 tablespoons soy sauce (low sodium)
- One tablespoon of Dijon mustard.
- 2 garlic cloves, minced
- One teaspoon honey (optional)
- 1/4 teaspoon black pepper.
- 1/2 teaspoon dried thyme.

Directions:

1. Prepare the marinade: - In a small mixing bowl, combine balsamic vinegar, soy sauce, Dijon mustard, garlic, honey (if using), black pepper, and thyme.

2. Marinate the Chicken: - Place the chicken thighs in a shallow dish or sealable bag. Pour the marinade over the chicken, making sure it's thoroughly coated.
Marinate for at least 15 minutes (up to 2 hours in the fridge for a more robust flavor).

3. To cook the chicken, heat a non-stick skillet over medium-high heat. Remove the chicken from the marinade and set aside the marinade for the glaze.
Cook the chicken thighs for 4-5 minutes per side, or until golden brown and fully cooked (165°F/74°C internal temperature).

4. Prepare the Glaze: - Simmer the reserved marinade in a skillet over medium heat until it thickens into a glaze (about 3-4 minutes).

5. Serve: Drizzle balsamic glaze on chicken thighs and serve immediately.

Health Benefits:

- **Rich Flavor, Low Fat:** Chicken thighs are tasty and contain healthy fats while being lean.
- **Gut Health**: Balsamic vinegar includes probiotics, which help digestion.
- **Balanced Nutrition:** The glaze provides a touch of sweetness without adding extra calories.

Tips:

➢ **Perfect Glaze:** Reduce the glaze slowly to achieve a rich, sticky consistency.
➢ **Side suggestions:** Serve with roasted Brussels sprouts or quinoa for a full dinner.
➢ **Alternative Protein:** This glaze pairs beautifully with fish or pork tenderloin.

Both recipes are versatile, healthy, and flavorful, making them great options for your zero-point lifestyle!

Chicken and Vegetable Skillet Stir-Fry

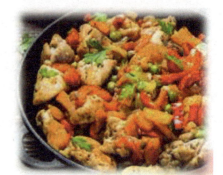

Prep Time: 10 minutes

Cooking Time: 15 minutes.

Total Time: 25 minutes.
Servings: 4

Ingredients:

- 1 lb (450 g) boneless, skinless chicken breasts cut into thin strips
- One tablespoon of olive oil (optional for nonstick pans)
- Two cups of broccoli florets
- 1 cup red bell pepper, sliced
- 1 cup sliced zucchini.
- 1 cup snap peas.
- 1/4 cup of low-sodium soy sauce.
- 1 tbsp. fresh ginger minced
- 2 garlic cloves, minced
- 1 tsp. corn-starch (optional, to thicken the sauce)
- One-quarter cup water

Directions:

1. Prepare the ingredients by slicing the chicken and veggies into bite-sized pieces.

2. To cook the chicken, prepare a large nonstick pan or wok over medium-high heat. Cook the chicken strips for 5-6 minutes, turning periodically, until thoroughly cooked and gently browned. Remove from the skillet and put aside.

3. Cook the Vegetables: In the same skillet, add the broccoli, bell pepper, zucchini, and snap peas. Stir-fry for 5-7 minutes, until the veggies are soft and crisp.

4. Make the Sauce: In a small bowl, combine the soy sauce, ginger, garlic, and cornstarch (if using). Add water to make a smooth sauce.

5. Combine and Serve: Return the chicken to the skillet and pour the sauce over it. Stir carefully to ensure that everything is coated equally. Cook for 2-3 minutes, until the sauce thickens slightly. Serve hot as is, or with cauliflower rice for a low-carb alternative.

Health Benefits:

- **High in Protein:** Chicken contains essential amino acids for muscle repair and energy.
- **Nutrient-dense vegetables:** Broccoli, snap peas, and peppers are high in vitamins, antioxidants, and fiber.

➤ **Low-Calorie Meal:** This dish is light and healthy thanks to the minimal amount of added fat.

Tips:

➤ **Customize the Vegetables:** Use any mix of veggies you have on hand, including carrots, mushrooms, and bok choy.
➤ **Increase Heat:** For a spicy kick, sprinkle with red pepper flakes or a splash of Sriracha.
➤ **Make it Meal Prep Friendly:** Refrigerate individual servings for up to 4 days.

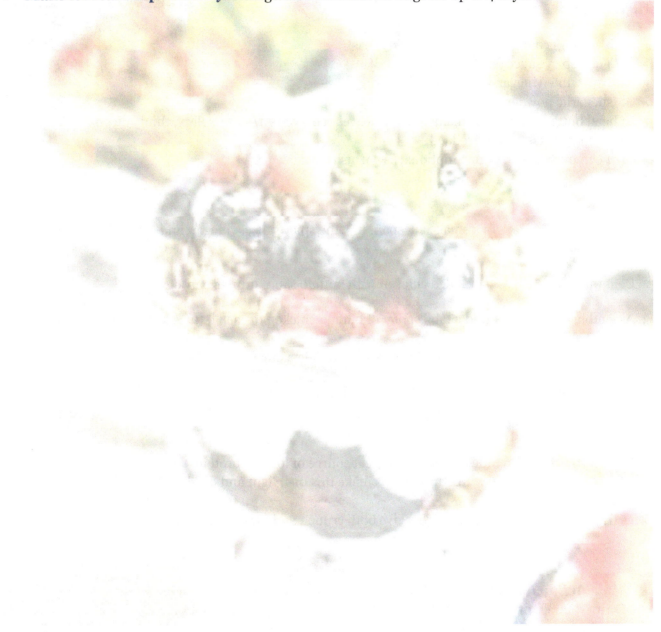

Buffalo Style Chicken Lettuce Wraps

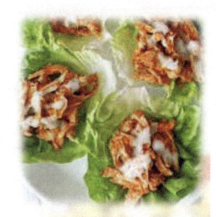

Prep Time: 10 minutes.
Cook Time: 10 minutes
Total Time: 20 minutes
Servings: 4 (8 wraps)

Ingredients:

- 1 lb. (450 g) cooked, shredded chicken breast
- 1/4 cup spicy sauce (such as Frank's RedHot)
- 2 tbsp. white vinegar
- 1 tsp. garlic powder
- 1 head butter lettuce or romaine lettuce, leaves removed - 1/2 cup celery, thinly diced
- 1/2 cup carrots, finely shredded
- 1/4 cup plain Greek yogurt (optional as garnish)

Directions:

1. Make Buffalo Sauce: - In a small saucepan, mix the spicy sauce, vinegar, and garlic powder. Heat on low heat until warm.

2. Coat the Chicken: Toss shredded chicken with buffalo sauce until evenly covered.

3. Assemble the Wraps: - Add a tablespoon of buffalo chicken to each lettuce leaf. Garnish with chopped celery and shredded carrots.
If preferred, top with a dollop of Greek yogurt to provide a creamy contrast.

4. Serve: Place wraps on a plate and serve immediately.

Health Benefits:

- **Lean Protein:** Shredded chicken is a great source of low-fat protein.
- **Low-Carb Alternative**: Lettuce wraps make this dish light and devoid of manufactured carbohydrates.
- **High in Fiber:** Celery and carrots give both crunch and nutritional fiber.

Tips:

- **Make It Spicier**: Add more hot sauce or cayenne pepper for a spicy kick.
- **Dairy-Free Option:** Omit the yogurt or substitute a plant-based option.
- **Meal preparation:** Preserve the buffalo chicken separately and assemble the wraps just before serving to preserve the lettuce crisp.

Both dishes are delectable, fast to prepare, and ideal for your zero-point weight-loss journey!

CHAPTER SIX

Vegetable Sides

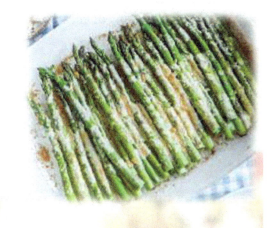

Roasted Garlic and Parmesan Asparagus

Prep Time: 5 minutes

Cooking Time: 15 minutes

Total Time: 2minutes

Servings: 4

Ingredients:

- ➢ 1 lb. (450 g) fresh asparagus, trimmed
- ➢ 2 garlic cloves, minced
- ➢ 1 tsp. olive oil spray (optional for nonstick).
- ➢ 2 tablespoons grated parmesan cheese.
- ➢ 1/4 teaspoon salt.
- ➢ 1/4 teaspoon black pepper.
- ➢ 1/2 tsp. lemon zest (optional as garnish)

Directions:

1. Preheat the oven to 400°F (200°C). Line a baking sheet with parchment paper or gently coat with olive oil spray.

2. Prepare asparagus: - Rinse the asparagus and clip off any rough ends. Arrange the asparagus stalks in a single layer on the prepared baking sheet.

3. To season the asparagus, sprinkle with chopped garlic, salt, and black pepper. Lightly spritz with olive oil to increase crispness.

4. Roast the Asparagus: Roast in a preheated oven for 12-15 minutes, until tender and slightly crispy at the tips.

5. Add Parmesan: - While still hot, sprinkle grated parmesan cheese over the asparagus. Allow the cheese to melt slightly.

6. To serve, transfer to a dish and garnish with lemon zest for a zesty touch (optional).

Health Benefits:

➤ **Rich in Vitamins:** Asparagus has high levels of vitamins A, C, E, K, and folate.
➤ **Low-Calorie Side:** This meal is low in calories yet full of taste.
➤ **Antioxidant Boost:** Garlic and Parmesan provide antioxidants and important minerals.

Tips:

➤ **Cooking Consistency:** Use asparagus spears of equal thickness for consistent cooking.
➤ **Add a twist:** Sprinkle with red pepper flakes for a spicy bite, or drizzle with balsamic glaze to add depth.
➤ **Perfect Pairing:** Serve with grilled chicken, fish, or a vegetarian main course.

This roasted garlic and parmesan asparagus recipe is a flexible and beautiful side dish that will complement any dinner.

Mediterranean Grilled Vegetable Platter

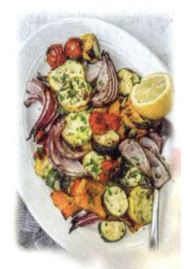

Prep Time: 10 minutes

Cooking Time: 15 minutes.

Total Time: 25 minutes.
Servings: 4

Ingredient:

- ➤ Slice one big zucchini and one large eggplant into 1/4-inch rounds.
- ➤ One red bell pepper, sliced into big pieces
- ➤ one yellow bell pepper, sliced into big strips
- ➤ One cup cherry tomatoes.
- ➤ One red onion, cut into thick rings
- ➤ 2 tablespoons lemon juice.
- ➤ 1 teaspoon olive oil spray.
- ➤ Add 2 tsp. dried oregano and 2 chopped garlic cloves.
- ➤ Add salt and black pepper to taste.
- ➤ Optional garnishes: fresh parsley or crumbled feta cheese.

Directions:

1. Preheat the Grill: - Set an outdoor grill or grill pan to medium-high heat.

2. Prepare the Veggies: - Place the zucchini, eggplant, bell peppers, cherry tomatoes, and onion in a large bowl.
Drizzle with lemon juice, and then gently spray with olive oil and season with oregano, minced garlic, salt, and pepper. Toss to coat evenly.

3. Grill the veggies: Grill veggies in batches, flipping regularly, until soft and with obvious grill marks (usually 2-3 minutes per side for most vegetables).
To avoid dropping through the grates, skewer or cook cherry tomatoes in a grill basket.

4. Assemble the plate: - Place the grilled veggies on a big plate. Garnish with fresh parsley or crumbled feta cheese, if preferred.

5. Serve: Serve warm or at room temperature with a side of hummus or tzatziki to dip.

Health Benefits:

- ➢ **Rich in Nutrients:** Fresh veggies include fiber, vitamins, and antioxidants.
- ➢ **Low Calorie and Filling:** Ideal for weight control and satiety.
- ➢ **Heart-Healthy:** Mediterranean-inspired flavors improve cardiovascular health.

Tips:

- ➢ **Customize Veggies:** Include mushrooms, asparagus, or other seasonal veggies in the mix.
- ➢ **Flavor Boost: Marinate** the veggies in the lemon-oregano mixture for 15 minutes before cooking.
- ➢ **Meal Prep-Friendly:** Grill in advance and keep in the refrigerator for up to 3 days.

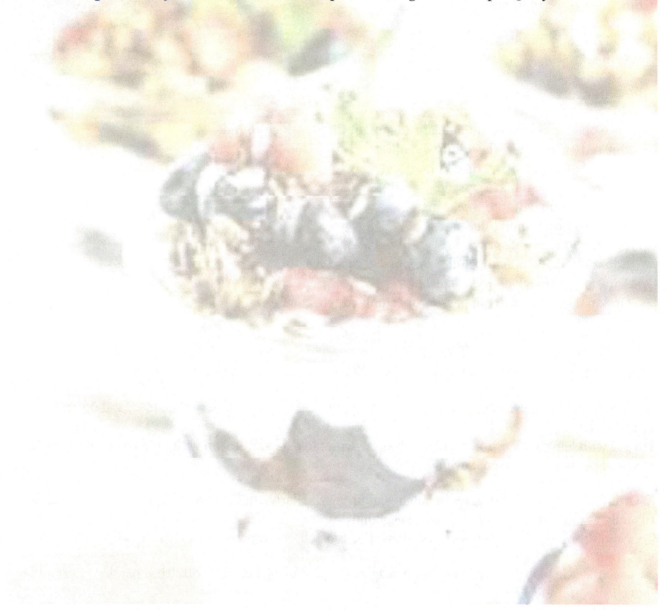

Spicy Cauliflower "Wings"

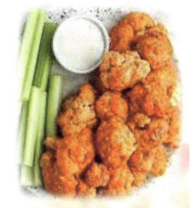

Prep Time: 10 minutes

Cooking Time: 30 minutes

Total Time: 40 minutes.
Servings: 4

Ingredients:

- 1 medium head of cauliflower, chopped into bite-sized florets
- 1/2 cup spicy sauce (such as Frank's Red-hot).
- Two tablespoons of white vinegar.
- One teaspoon of garlic powder.
- One teaspoon of smoked paprika.
- 1/4 tsp cayenne pepper (optional for added spice).
- Cooking Spray

Directions:

1. Preheat the oven to 425°F (220°C). Line a baking sheet with parchment paper or gently coat with cooking spray.

2. Prepare the Cauliflower: - Spread cauliflower florets equally on a baking sheet.

3. Make the Sauce: In a small saucepan, mix together the spicy sauce, vinegar, garlic powder, smoked paprika, and cayenne pepper. Cook over low heat for 2-3 minutes, stirring periodically.

4. To bake the cauliflower, lightly coat it with cooking spray. Bake for 20 minutes and turn halfway through.

5. Toss in Sauce: Remove cauliflower from oven and toss with spicy sauce until evenly covered. Return to the oven for another ten minutes to caramelize.

6. Serve: Arrange cauliflower "wings" on a dish. Serve immediately, accompanied by celery sticks and ranch or blue cheese dressing (optional).

Health Benefits:

- **Low in Calories:** A filling snack without the fat and calories of fried wings.
- **High in Fiber:** Cauliflower improves digestion and intestinal health.
- **Packed with Flavor:** Spices increase metabolism and provide antioxidants.

Tips:

➢ **Air Fryer Option**: Cook cauliflower florets at 400°F (200°C) for 15-20 minutes to achieve a crispier texture.
➢ **Adjust the Spice Level**: For less heat, reduce the cayenne pepper or substitute a milder hot sauce.
➢ **Meal preparation:** Make the sauce and cut the cauliflower ahead of time for easy assembling.

Both recipes are tasty, flexible, and make excellent contributions to any meal or party!

Zesty Lemon Green Beans

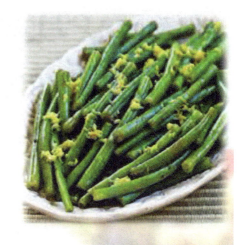

Prep Time: 5 minutes.

Cooking Time: 10 minutes

Total Time: 15 minutes.
Serving: 4

Ingredient:

- 1 lb (450 g) fresh, trimmed green beans
- One tablespoon of lemon juice.
  Add 1 tsp lemon zest and 2 chopped garlic cloves.
- 1/4 teaspoon salt.
- 1/4 teaspoon black pepper.
- 1 tsp olive oil spray (optional for non-stick).
- Optional garnishes: fresh parsley or sliced almonds.

Directions:

1. Prepare Green Beans: - Rinse and cut the ends.

2. Blanch Green Beans: Heat a big saucepan of water to a boil. Add the green beans and blanch for 3-4 minutes, or until they are brilliant green and crispy crisp. Drain and immediately transfer to an ice bath to halt the cooking.

3. To sauté the green beans, prepare a non-stick pan over medium heat. Spray gently with olive oil. Add the minced garlic and cook for 30 seconds, or until fragrant.

4. Add lemon and seasoning. Combine the blanched green beans, lemon juice, and zest. Stir well to get a uniform coating. Season with salt and black pepper. Cook for 2-3 minutes, until well heated.

5. Serve: Transfer to a serving plate and decorate with fresh parsley or slivered almonds as preferred.

Health Benefits:

- **High in Nutrients:** Green beans include vitamins A, C, and K, as well as dietary fiber.
- **Low in Calories:** A light yet filling side dish that promotes weight reduction.
- **Antioxidant Boost:** Lemon zest and garlic provide antioxidants to your food.

Tips:

- **Add Crunch:** Sprinkle with toasted sesame or pumpkin seeds for added texture.
- **Increase Flavor:** Add a sprinkle of red pepper flakes for a spice boost.
- **Meal Prep-Friendly:** Keep in an airtight container for up to three days.

CHAPTER SEVEN

VEGETARIAN MAINS

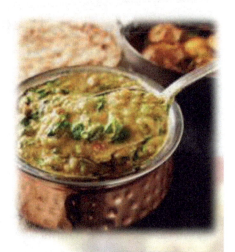

Lentil and Spinach Curry

Prep Time: 10 minutes

Cooking Time: 25 minutes.

Total Time: 35 minutes.
Servings: 4

Ingredients:

- 1 cup washed, dry red lentils.
- Four cups of veggie broth or water
- One tablespoon curry powder.
- 1 tsp ground cumin, 1/2 tsp turmeric.
- 1/2 teaspoon smoked paprika.
- Dice one medium onion and mince three garlic cloves.
- Grate 1 inch of ginger. - Use 1 can (14 oz) chopped tomatoes.
- Roughly cut 4 cups of fresh spinach leaves. - Season with salt and black pepper to taste. Optional garnish: Fresh cilantro and a squeeze of lime

Directions:

1. Prepare the Lentils: Rinse the lentils under cold water until the water runs clear.

2. Sauté the Aromatics: Heat a large pot over medium heat. Add the diced onion and cook until softened (3-4 minutes). Add the garlic and ginger, cooking for another minute until fragrant.

3. Add Spices: Stir in the curry powder, cumin, turmeric, and smoked paprika. Cook for 1 minute, stirring constantly to toast the spices.

4. Cook the Lentils: Add the rinsed lentils, diced tomatoes, and vegetable broth to the pot. Stir to combine and bring to a boil. Reduce the heat to low, cover, and simmer for 20 minutes, stirring occasionally, until the lentils are tender and the mixture is thickened.

5. Add the Spinach: Stir in the chopped spinach and cook for 2-3 minutes, until wilted.

6. Season and Serve: Taste and adjust seasoning with salt and black pepper. Serve hot, garnished with fresh cilantro and a squeeze of lime, if desired.

Health Benefits:

➢ **High in Protein and Fiber:** Lentils provide plant-based protein and promote digestion.
➢ **Rich in Antioxidants:** Spinach and turmeric add antioxidants that boost immunity and reduce inflammation.
➢ **Heart-Healthy:** Low in saturated fat and cholesterol while packed with essential nutrients like iron and folate.

Tips:

➢ **Make it Creamy:** Stir in 1/4 cup of unsweetened coconut milk for a richer curry.
➢ **Bulk it Up:** Add diced sweet potatoes or carrots for extra heartiness.
➢ **Meal Prep:** This curry tastes even better the next day, making it a great meal prep option. Store in the fridge for up to 4 days or freeze for up to 3 months.

This lentil and spinach curry is a satisfying, nutrient-packed meal that's as delicious as it is healthy!

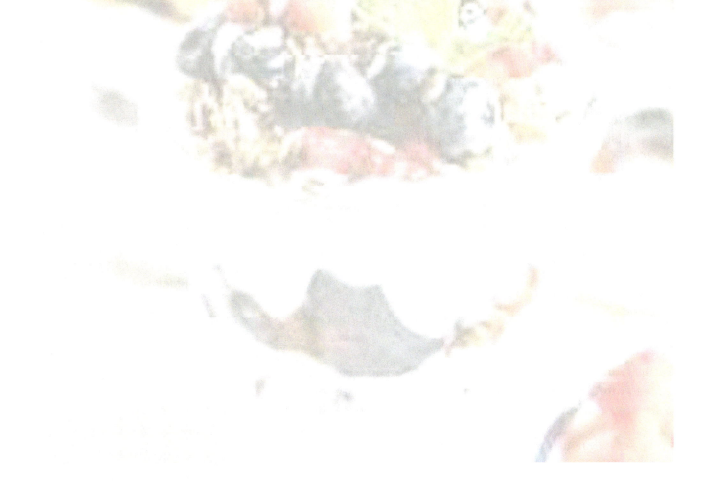

Stuffed Bell Peppers with Quinoa and Chickpeas

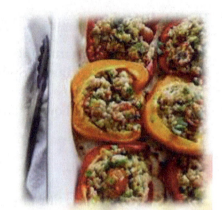

Prep Time: 15 minutes

Cooking Time: 30 minutes

Total Time: 45 minutes.
Servings: 4

Ingredients:

➢ 4 big bell peppers (any color), tops chopped off and seeds removed
➢ 1 cup cooked quinoa
➢ 1 cup canned chickpeas, drained and rinsed

Ingredients:

➢ (Fresh or canned).
➢ 1/2 cup chopped spinach or kale.
➢ 1 tsp ground cumin, 1/2 tsp smoked paprika.
➢ 1/2 teaspoon garlic powder.
➢ 1/4 tsp salt and 1/4 tsp black pepper.
➢ Optional garnishes: chopped parsley and a sprinkle of lemon juice

Directions:

1. Preheat the oven to 375°F (190°C).

2. Prepare the Filling: - In a large mixing bowl, mix together the cooked quinoa, chickpeas, diced tomatoes, chopped spinach, cumin, smoked paprika, garlic powder, salt, and black pepper. Mix well.

3. Stuff the Peppers: - Fill each bell pepper with quinoa and chickpea mixture, carefully pressing to pack.

4. Bake the Peppers: Place the stuffed peppers in a baking dish. To prevent sticking, add about 1/4 cup of water to the bottom of the dish. Cover the dish with foil and bake for 25 min.
   Remove the foil and bake for an additional 5 minutes until the tops are slightly browned.

5. To serve, garnish with chopped parsley and a drizzle of lemon juice.

Health Benefits:

➢ **High in Fiber:** Chickpeas and quinoa improve digestive health and keep you fuller for longer.
➢ **Full of Vitamins:** Bell peppers are abundant in vitamin C and antioxidants.

➢ **Plant-Based Protein**: Excellent vegetarian source of protein and necessary amino acids.

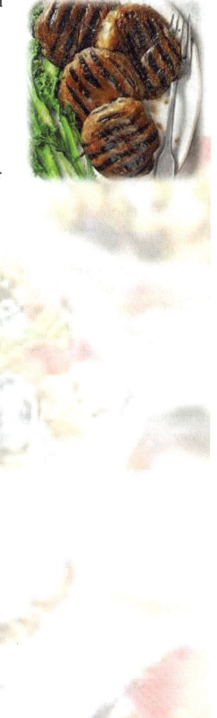

Tips:

➢ **Customize the Filling:** Add more vegetables such as zucchini, corn, or shredded carrots for diversity.
➢ **Spice It Up:** For extra heat, add a pinch of red pepper flakes.
➢ **Dinner Prep:** These stuffed peppers reheat well and are ideal for dinner preparation.

Grilled Portobello Mushroom "Steaks"

Prep Time: 10 minutes

Cooking Time: 10 minutes

Total Time: 20 minutes.
Servings: 4

Ingredients:

➤ 4 large Portobello mushrooms, stems removed
➤ 2 tbsp balsamic vinegar
➤ 1 tbsp soy sauce (low sodium)
➤ One teaspoon olive oil (optional)
➤ One teaspoon of garlic powder.
➤ 1/2 teaspoon smoked paprika.
➤ 1/4 teaspoon black pepper.
➤ Optional garnishes: fresh thyme or parsley

Directions:

1. Prepare the marinade: - In a small mixing bowl, combine balsamic vinegar, soy sauce, olive oil (if using), garlic powder, smoked paprika, and black pepper.

2. Marinate the mushrooms: Put the Portobello mushrooms in a shallow dish and pour the marinade over them. Allow them to sit for at least 10 minutes, flipping midway to coat both sides.

3. Heat the Grill: - Preheat a grill or grill pan to medium heat.

4. Grill the mushrooms. Cook the mushrooms on the grill, gill side down, for 4-5 minutes. Flip and heat for a further 4-5 minutes, or until tender and slightly charred.

5. To serve, arrange the mushrooms on a plate and garnish with fresh thyme or parsley.

Health Benefits:

➤ **Low-Calorie and Nutrient-Rich**: Portobello mushrooms have significant levels of potassium, selenium, and B vitamins.
➤ **Heart Healthy:** Contains no cholesterol and little saturated fat.
➤ **Antioxidant Powerhouse:** Balsamic vinegar and mushrooms contain antioxidants that fight inflammation.

Tips:

➤ Pair with roasted veggies or a side salad for a full dinner.
➤ Increase Flavor: Brush with more marinade while grilling for added intensity.
➤ Versatile Option: Grilled mushrooms can be used as burger patties or sliced into wraps and salads.

Both recipes are savory, satisfying, and great for a healthy vegetarian supper!

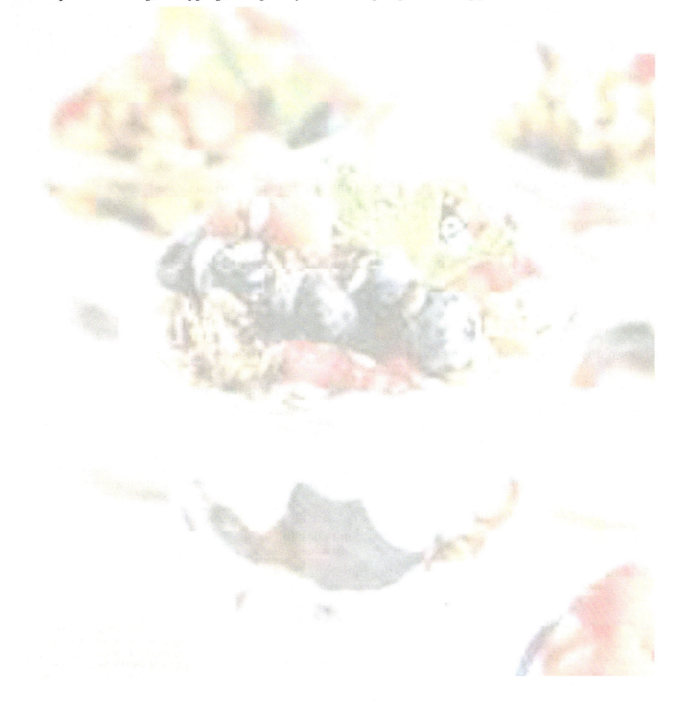

"Zucchini Noodles with Tomato Basil Sauce"

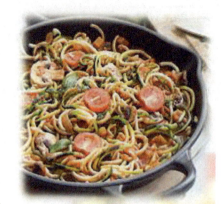

Prep Time: 10 minutes

Cooking Time: 10 minutes

Total Tim: 20 minutes.
Servings: 4

Ingredients:

- 4 medium zucchini spiralized into noodles.
- Two cups of diced fresh tomatoes (or one 14-ounce can of crushed tomatoes)
- Mince 2 garlic cloves. - Finely cut 1 small onion.
- 1/4 cup freshly cut basil leaves.
- One teaspoon olive oil (optional)
- Season with salt and black pepper to taste. - Add optional garnishes. Grated parmesan cheese (if desired, modify points appropriately).

Directions:

1. Prepare zucchini noodles using a spiralizer or julienne peeler. Set aside.

2. Cook the Sauce: Place a skillet on medium heat. If you're using olive oil, add it to the skillet. Sauté the onion and garlic for 2-3 minutes, until they are tender and fragrant.
Stir in the diced tomatoes and simmer for 5-7 minutes, stirring periodically. Season with salt and pepper.

3. Add Basil: Stir in chopped basil and simmer for another minute. Remove from heat.

4. Cook the Zucchini Noodles: In a separate skillet, briskly sauté the zucchini noodles for 2-3 minutes, until just tender but firm. To avoid sogginess, don't cook too long.

5. Combine and Serve: Toss zucchini noodles in tomato basil sauce. Serve immediately, topped with extra fresh basil or parmesan if desired.

Health Benefits:

- **Low-Calorie Alternative:** Zucchini noodles are a low-calorie pasta option that can help reduce calorie intake dramatically.
- **Vitamin-Rich:** Zucchini is high in vitamin C and potassium, whereas tomatoes include lycopene, an antioxidant.
- **Digestive Health:** The meal is abundant in fiber, which improves gut health.

CHAPTER EIGHT

SNACKS AND APPETIZERS

Cucumber and Hummus Roll-ups

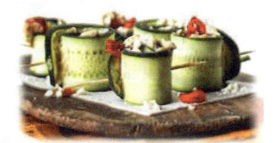

Prep Time: 10 minutes.
Cooking time: None
Total Time: 10 minutes
Servings: 4 (about 16 roll-ups).

Ingredients:

- One large cucumber finely sliced lengthwise with a mandoline or vegetable peeler.
- 1/2 cup hummus, either store-bought or homemade.
- 1/4 cup shredded carrots.
- 1/4 cup red bell pepper, thinly cut into strips
- 2 tablespoons of chopped fresh parsley or cilantro (optional)
- Add salt and black pepper to taste.

Directions:

1. Prepare cucumber slices: Wash the cucumber and cut it lengthwise into thin ribbons with a mandolin or vegetable peeler. To eliminate any extra moisture, pat dry with a paper towel.

2. Spread the Hummus: Place each cucumber slices flat on a clean surface and spread a thin coating of hummus over it.

3. Fillings: - Add shredded carrots and a strip of red bell pepper to one end of each cucumber slice.

4. Roll them Up: Begin by wrapping the cucumber slice tightly around the bell pepper strip, forming a little spiral. Secure with a toothpick if necessary.

5. Season and Serve: - Sprinkle roll-ups with fresh parsley or cilantro, then season with salt and pepper as desired. Serve immediately.

Health Benefits:

- **Hydration Boost**: Cucumber's high water content helps keep you hydrated.
- **Nutrition-Rich:** Contains vitamins A, C, and E from veggies.
- **Low Calorie and Satisfying:** Hummus contains fiber and protein, which helps to satisfy hunger.

Tips:

➤ **Homemade Hummus:** Blend chickpeas, garlic, tahini, lemon juice, and water for a fresh, preservative-free choice.

➤ **Customize the Fillings:** For more variation, add thinly sliced vegetables such as zucchini, radish, or avocado.

➤ **Make ahead:** These roll-ups can be prepared a few hours ahead of time and refrigerated.

Cucumber and hummus roll-ups are a nutritious and colorful complement to any snack spread or appetizer tray.

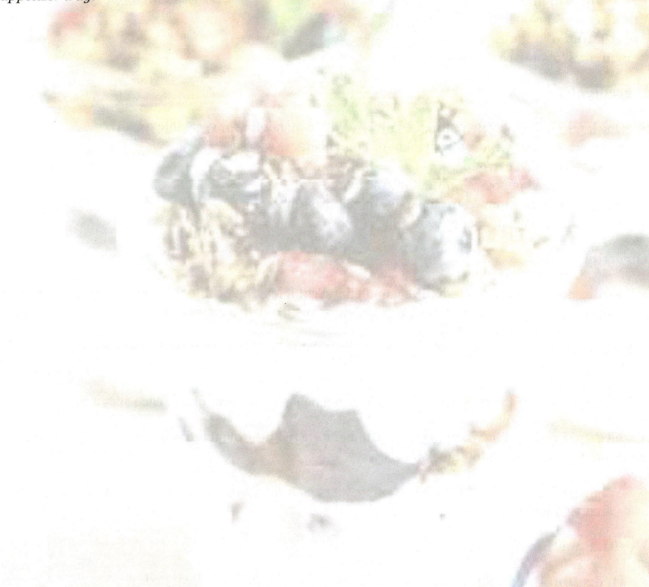

Peppery Roasted Chickpeas

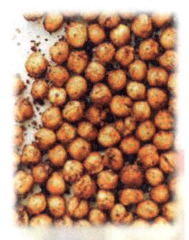

Prep Time: 10 minutes

Cooking Time: 25 minutes.

Total Time: 35 minutes.
Servings: 4

Ingredients:

➤ One can (15 oz) of drained and washed chickpeas
➤ 1 tablespoon olive oil (optional, for added crispiness)
➤ One teaspoon of chili powder
➤ 1/2 teaspoon smoked paprika.
➤ 1/4 teaspoon garlic powder.
➤ 1/4 tsp cayenne pepper (optional for added heat).
➤ Add salt and black pepper to taste.

Directions:

1. Preheat the oven to 400°F (200°C).

2. Prepare chickpeas: Drain and rinse the chickpeas, then pat them dry with a paper towel. This step is critical to having them crispy!

3. Season the chickpeas: - In a bowl, combine the chickpeas, olive oil (if using), chili powder, smoked paprika, garlic powder, cayenne pepper, salt, and black pepper. Make sure the chickpeas are covered evenly.

4. Roast: - Place chickpeas in a single layer on a baking sheet. Bake for 20-25 minutes, stirring halfway, until golden brown and crispy.

5. Chill and Serve: Allow the chickpeas to chill for a few minutes before serving. They will become even crisper as they cool.

Health Benefits:

➤ **High in Protein and Fiber:** Chickpeas provide plant-based protein and fiber, promoting satiety and digestive health.
➤ **Low in Calories:** These roasted chickpeas are a crunchy, delicious snack that is without the additional calories found in regular chips.
➤ **High in Antioxidants:** Spices such as chili powder and paprika have antioxidant properties.

Greek Yogurt and Herb Dip for Veggies

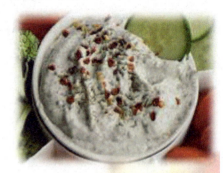

Prep Time: 5 minutes.
Cooking Time: None

Total Time: 5 min
Servings: 4

Ingredients:

➤ 1 cup plain Greek yogurt (fat-free)
➤ 1 tbsp fresh dill chopped (or 1 tsp dried dill)
➤ 1 tablespoon fresh parsley, chopped
➤ One teaspoon of garlic powder.
➤ One tablespoon of lemon juice.
➤ Season to taste with salt and pepper.
➤ Serve with fresh veggies for dipping, such as carrots, cucumbers, bell peppers, and celery.

Directions:

1. Prepare the dip: - In a small mixing bowl, combine Greek yogurt, dill, parsley, garlic powder, lemon juice, salt, and pepper. Stir until smooth and fully integrated.

2. Serve: - Serve immediately with fresh vegetables like carrot sticks, cucumber slices, bell pepper strips, or celery.

Health Benefits:

➤ **High in Protein:** Greek yogurt contains high levels of protein, which encourage muscle building and satiety.
➤ **Gut Health:** Greek yogurt contains probiotics, which help maintain a healthy gut.
➤ **Full of Vitamins**: Fresh herbs like parsley and dill contain vitamins A, C, and K, while vegetables provide fiber, antioxidants, and hydration.

Tip:

➤ **Make Ahead**: Refrigerate the dip for up to 3 days.
➤ **Include Zing:** For a hotter dip, add a splash of hot sauce or red pepper flakes.
➤ **Customize:** For more taste, add herbs such as chives, thyme, or tarragon.

Both of these snacks are light, nutritional, and quite gratifying! They'll keep you full and invigorated while helping you stick to your zero-point meal plan.

Mini Caprese Skewers

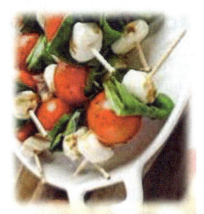

Prep Time: 10 minutes.
Cooking Time: None.

Total Time: 10 min
Servings: 4

Ingredients:

➢ 1 pint cherry tomatoes - 1 cup fresh mozzarella balls (bocconcini or ciliegine).
➢ 1/4 cup fresh basil leaves.
➢ One tablespoon of balsamic vinegar.
➢ Season to taste with salt and black pepper. - Drizzle with 1 tsp olive oil (optional).
➢ Wooden skewers, toothpicks

Directions:

1. Prepare the skewers: - Attach a cherry tomato, a mozzarella ball, and a fresh basil leaf to each skewer or toothpick. Repeat until all ingredients have been used up.

2. Season: Drizzle skewers with balsamic vinegar and olive oil (optional). Season with salt and pepper to taste.

3. Serve: Place the skewers on a dish and serve immediately or chill until ready to serve.

Health Benefits:

➢ **Rich in Protein and Calcium:** Mozzarella contains critical nutrients for bone and muscular health.
➢ **Rich in Antioxidants:** Tomatoes contain lycopene, an antioxidant that promotes heart health.
➢ **Low Calorie:** These skewers are a nutritious, low-calorie snack made with fresh, natural ingredients.

Tips:

➢ **Make Ahead:** Prepare these skewers ahead of time and refrigerate for simple serving.
➢ **Customize**: For added flavor, drizzle with pesto or sprinkle with crushed red pepper flakes.
➢ **Use Skewer Alternatives:** For a less formal presentation, place the components on a dish without skewers.

Deviled Eggs with a Twist

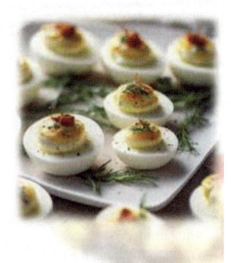

Prep Time: 10 minutes.
Cook Time: 10 minutes
Total Time: 20 minutes
Servings: 4 (equal 8 deviled eggs)

Ingredients:

➤ Four big eggs.
➤ 2 tablespoons plain Greek yogurt (non-fat).
➤ 1 tsp Dijon mustard, 1 tsp apple cider vinegar.
➤ 1/4 teaspoon garlic powder.
➤ 1/4 teaspoon smoked paprika.
➤ Add salt and black pepper to taste.
➤ Fresh chives or parsley, diced (optional for garnish).

Directions:

1. Cook the Eggs: Put the eggs in a pot and cover with water. Bring to a boil, then reduce the heat to a simmer. Cook for 9–10 minutes. Remove the eggs from the pot and allow them to cool in cold water.

2. Prepare the Filling: - Peel the eggs and cut in half lengthwise. Remove the yolks and transfer them to a small mixing dish. Mash the yolks with a fork.
Mix in the Greek yogurt, Dijon mustard, apple cider vinegar, garlic powder, smoked paprika, salt, and pepper with the mashed yolks. Mix until smooth and creamy.

3. Fill the Eggs: Spoon or pipe the filling into the egg whites.

4. Garnish and Serve: Add fresh chives or parsley and smoked paprika for color. Serve immediately or chill until ready to enjoy.

Health Benefits:

➤ **High in Protein:** Eggs are a great source of protein, which helps with muscle repair and growth.
➤ **Gut-Friendly:** Greek yogurt contains probiotics, which promote digestive health.
➤ **Low-Calorie:** A healthier version of deviled eggs that does not use mayonnaise, lowering the calorie count while maintaining flavor.

Tips:

➤ **Add Flavor:** Add hot sauce or pickled jalapeños to the filling for a spicy kick.
➤ **Make Ahead:** These devilled eggs can be prepared a few hours ahead of time and refrigerated.
➤ **Customize:** To change up the flavor profile, add herbs like dill, tarragon, or chives to the filling.

CHAPTER NINE

STEWS AND SOUPS

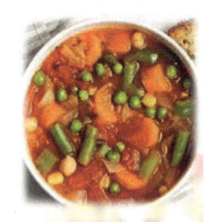

Hearty Vegetable Soup

Prep Time: 15 minutes

Cooking Time: 30 minutes

Total Time: 45 minutes.
Servings: 6

Ingredients:

- Sliced onion, minced garlic cloves, peeled and chopped carrots, and chopped celery stalks.
- 1 zucchini, diced
- 1 cup trimmed green beans, chopped into 1-inch pieces.
- 1 cup shredded cabbage.
- 1 can (14 oz) chopped tomatoes without added salt
- 6 cups vegetable broth (low sodium)
- Use 1 tsp dried thyme and 1 tsp dry oregano.
- 1/2 teaspoon smoked paprika.
- Add salt and black pepper to taste.
- Fresh parsley, chopped (to garnish)

Directions:

1. To sauté the aromatics, heat a large pot over medium heat. Sauté the onion and garlic for 2-3 minutes, until fragrant and tender.

2. Add the Vegetables: - Combine carrots, celery, zucchini, green beans, and cabbage. Cook for an additional 5 minutes, stirring occasionally.

3. To simmer the soup, combine diced tomatoes, vegetable broth, thyme, oregano, smoked paprika, salt, and pepper. Bring the soup to a boil, then reduce to a low heat and simmer for 20-25 minutes, until the veggies are soft.

4. Adjust Seasoning: Taste the soup and add salt and pepper as needed.

5. Serve: Ladle soup into dishes, garnish with fresh parsley, and serve hot.

Health Benefits:

➢ **Low-Calorie, Nutrient-Dense:** Packed with a variety of veggies, this soup is high in vitamins, minerals, and fiber.
➢ **Hydrating and Filling:** The broth-based soup hydrates you while making you feel full.
➢ **Heart-Healthy:** Low in salt and saturated fat, making it beneficial to heart health.

Tips:

➢ **Add Protein:** Add shredded chicken, tofu, or beans to make a heartier soup.
➢ **Customize the vegetables:** Use any vegetables you have on hand, including spinach, kale, and sweet potatoes.
➢ **Make ahead:** This soup tastes even better the second day, as the flavors mature. Refrigerate in an airtight container for up to 4 days, or freeze for up to 3 months.

This hearty vegetable soup is a good alternative for those following a zero-point meal plan. It's tasty, flexible, and simple to prepare—ideal for any time of year!

Chicken and Zoodle Soup

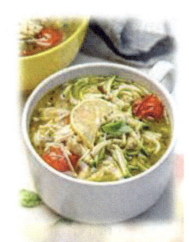

Prep Time: 15 minutes

Cooking Time: 25 minutes

Total Time: 40 minutes.
Servings: 4

Ingredients:

- ➤ One pound boneless, skinless chicken breast.
- ➤ Four cups of zucchini noodles (spiralized from two medium zucchini)
- ➤ one large carrot, peeled and sliced
- ➤ To prepare, chop 2 celery stalks, dice 1 small onion, and mince 2 garlic cloves.
- ➤ 6 cups chicken broth (low sodium)
- ➤ Add 1 tsp dried thyme, 1 tsp dried parsley, 1/2 tsp black pepper, and 1/2 tsp salt (optional).
- ➤ One tablespoon of fresh lemon juice (optional)

Directions:

1. To cook the chicken, bring chicken broth to a boil in a big pot. Add the chicken breast and decrease the heat to a simmer. Cover and heat for 10 to 12 minutes, or until the chicken is well cooked. Remove the chicken and set aside to cool.

2. Prepare the Vegetables: - In the same saucepan, add the carrots, celery, onion, and garlic. Simmer for 8-10 minutes, until the vegetables are soft.

3. Shred the Chicken: Use two forks to shred the chicken into bite-sized pieces after it has cooled.

4. Combine Ingredients: Return shredded chicken to the saucepan. Combine the zucchini noodles, thyme, parsley, salt, and pepper. Simmer for 3-5 minutes, until the zoodles are soft but not mushy.

5. Finish and Serve: - Add lemon juice (optional) for a fresh, tart finish. Serve hot.

Health Benefits:

- ➤ **Low in Carbs:** Replace regular pasta with zucchini noodles for a lighter, low-carb alternative.
- ➤ **High in Protein:** Chicken contains lean protein that keeps you satisfied and energized.
- ➤ **Immune Boosting:** Carrots, celery, and garlic are high in vitamins and antioxidants.

Tips:

- ➤ **Prepare Ahead**: To save time, spiralize the zucchini noodles and prepare the vegetables ahead of time.
- ➤ **Add More Greens:** Add spinach or kale for added nutrition.

Lentil and tomato stew

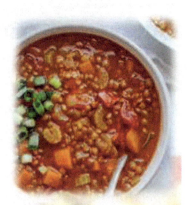

Prep Time: 10 minutes

Cooking Time: 35 minutes

Total Time: 45 minutes.
Servings: 4

Ingredients:

- 1 cup dried green or brown lentils, washed
- 1 can (14 oz) chopped tomatoes without added salt
- 4 cups vegetable broth (low sodium)
- one medium onion, diced
- 2 garlic cloves, minced
- two medium carrots, diced
- 1 teaspoon ground cumin.
- One teaspoon of smoked paprika.
- Add 1/2 tsp turmeric and 1/4 tsp chili flakes (optional).
- Add salt and black pepper to taste.
- Fresh cilantro, chopped (to garnish)

Directions:

1. To sauté the aromatics, heat a large pot over medium heat. Cook the onion and garlic for 2-3 minutes, or until tender and fragrant.

2. Cook the Base: - Combine chopped tomatoes, carrots, cumin, smoked paprika, turmeric, chili flakes (optional), and lentils. Stir to mix.

3. Simmer the stew. Add the veggie broth and bring to a boil. Reduce the heat to low and cook the stew for 25-30 minutes, or until the lentils are cooked. Stir occasionally.

4. Season and Serve: - Taste the stew and season with salt and pepper. Garnish with fresh cilantro and serve hot.

Health Benefits:

- **High in Fiber and Protein:** Lentils contain critical nutrients, aid digestion, and keep you fuller for longer.
- **High in Antioxidants:** Tomatoes and spices such as turmeric reduce inflammation and promote general health.
- **Heart-Healthy:** Low in saturated fat, high in plant-based protein.

Spicy Pumpkin Soup

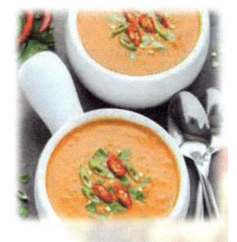

Prep Time: 10 minutes

Cooking Time: 25 minutes.

Total Time: 35 minutes.
Servings: 4

Ingredients:

➢ 4 cups pumpkin puree (homemade or canned, without extra sugar)
➢ Dice one medium onion and cut two garlic cloves.
➢ One tiny apple, peeled and diced
➢ 4 cups vegetable broth (low sodium)
➢ 1 tsp ground cumin, 1/2 tsp ground cinnamon.
➢ 1/4 teaspoon ground nutmeg.
➢ 1/4 teaspoon smoked paprika.
➢ Add salt and black pepper to taste.
➢ 1/4 cup of unsweetened almond milk (optional for creaminess).
➢ Fresh parsley or pumpkin seeds (as garnish)

Directions:

1. Sauté Aromatics: - Cook onion and garlic in a large pot over medium heat for 2-3 minutes, until aromatic.

2. Add Pumpkin and Apple: - Combine pumpkin puree and diced apple. Cook for a further 3-4 minutes, allowing the flavors to combine.

3. Add Broth and Spices: - Add the vegetable broth, cumin, cinnamon, nutmeg, smoked paprika, salt, and pepper. Heat the mixture to a boil, then reduce to a simmer. Cook for 15 minutes, stirring periodically.

4. Using an immersion blender, purée the soup until smooth. Alternatively, put the soup in a blender in batches and process carefully.

5. Optional: Add almond milk for creaminess.

6. To serve, ladle soup into bowls, decorate with fresh parsley or pumpkin seeds, and serve warm.

Health Benefits: Rich in Beta-Carotene: Pumpkin contains significant levels of vitamin A, which promotes eye health and immunity.

Low Calories: Despite its creamy texture, this soup is both light and low in calories.

Anti-Inflammatory: Spices such as cinnamon and paprika can help reduce inflammation.

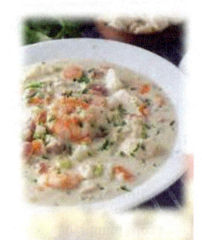

Seafood Chowder

Prep Time: 15 minutes

Cooking Time: 25 minutes

Total Time: 40 minutes.
Servings: 4

Ingredients: -

- 1 lb mixed seafood (shrimp, scallops, white fish) - 1 small onion, diced
- 2 celery stalks, chopped.
- One medium carrot, chopped.
- 1 garlic clove, minced
- 4 cups of fish or vegetable broth (low in sodium)
- One cup unsweetened almond milk.
- One large potato, peeled and diced (optional)
- Add 1 tsp dried thyme and 1/2 tsp smoky paprika.
- 1/4 teaspoon of cayenne pepper (optional)
- Add salt and black pepper to taste.
- Fresh parsley for garnish.

Directions:

1. In a large pot, sauté onion, celery, carrot, and garlic until softened (3-4 minutes).

2. Stir in the broth, thyme, smoked paprika, cayenne pepper (optional), salt, and black pepper. Bring to a boil.

3. Optional: Cook diced potato for 10-12 minutes, until cooked.

4. Add the fish: Reduce heat to a simmer and gently add the fish. Cook for 5-7 minutes, until the shrimp are pink and the fish flakes easily.

5. To add creaminess, stir in almond milk and cook for 2-3 minutes.

6. Serve: Ladle soup into bowls, sprinkle with fresh parsley, and serve warm.

Health Benefits:

- **High in Lean Protein:** Seafood is a rich source of protein and omega-3 fatty acids.
- **Heart-Healthy:** Low in saturated fat, high in important nutrients.

➤ **Full of Vitamins:** Packed with vegetables for extra fiber and vitamins.

Tips: Vary the Seafood: Try clams, crab, or mussels for unique flavors.
Make it dairy-free: Use almond milk for a creamy yet light texture.

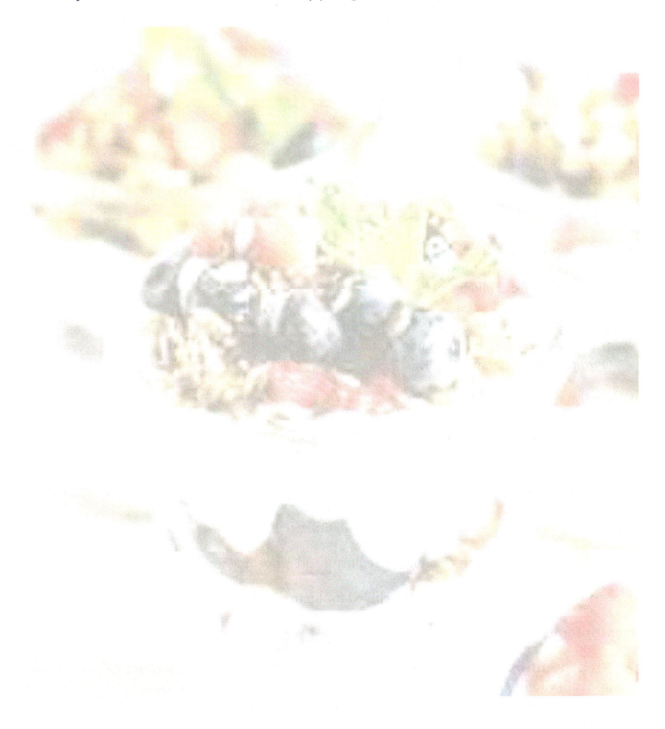

CHAPTER TEN

DESSERT

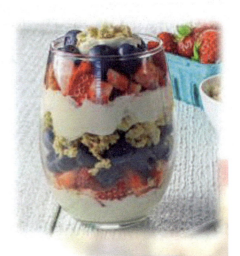

Berry and Yogurt Parfait

Prep Time: 10 minutes.
Cooking Time: None.

Total Time: 10 min
Servings: 2

Ingredients:

- 1 cup non-fat plain Greek yogurt.
- 1/2 cup fresh, sliced strawberries
- Half a cup of fresh blueberries
- 1/2 cup fresh raspberries.
- 1/2 teaspoon of pure vanilla essence (optional)
- 1/4 teaspoon of ground cinnamon (optional)
- One sprig of fresh mint for garnish.

Directions:

1. Prepare the yogurt: - In a small bowl, combine the Greek yogurt, vanilla essence, and cinnamon (if using). This provides a sense of sweetness and spice.

2. Place the Parfait: In a transparent glass or parfait dish, place roughly 2 teaspoons of yogurt.
Add a layer of mixed berries, distributing them evenly.
Continue layering until all of the ingredients are utilized, then top with berries.

3. Garnish: Add a sprig of fresh mint for a colorful and refreshing touch.

4. Serve: Can be served immediately or chilled for up to 1 hour.

Health Benefits:

- **Rich in Antioxidants:** Berries include vitamins and antioxidants that promote immune health and skin vitality.
- **High in Protein**: Greek yogurt has more protein, which helps you stay fuller for longer.
- **Low in Calories**: This dessert is both light and tasty, making it ideal for weight management.

This berry and yogurt parfait is simple to make, gorgeous to serve, and a delicious way to indulge without feeling guilty!

Baked Cinnamon Apples

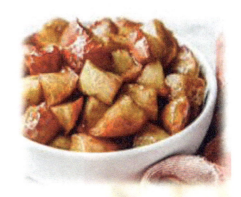

Prep Time: 10 minutes

Cooking Time: 25 minutes.

Total Time: 35 minutes.
Servings: 4

Ingredients:

➢ 4 medium apples (Gala or Fuji)
➢ One teaspoon of ground cinnamon
➢ 1/4 teaspoon ground nutmeg.
➢ 1/2 teaspoon of pure vanilla extract.
➢ Juice from 1/2 lemon.
➢ One-quarter cup water

Directions:

1. Preheat the oven to 375°F (190°C).

2. Prepare the Apples: - Wash and core the apples, leaving the bottom intact for the filling. Optional: peel the top third of each apple.

3. Season the Apples - In a small bowl, combine cinnamon, nutmeg, and vanilla extract. Rub the mixture into the apples.

4. Arrange in a baking dish. Put the apples in a baking dish. Drizzle the apples with lemon juice and pour the water into the dish.

5. Bake: Cover the dish with aluminum foil and bake for 20-25 minutes, or until apples are soft but not mushy.

6. Serve: Serve warm with a dollop of nonfat Greek yogurt for extra smoothness.

Health Benefits:

➢ **High in Fiber:** Apples promote digestive health and help you feel fuller.
➢ **Naturally sweetened:** With no added sugar, this is a healthier dessert option.
➢ **Packed with Antioxidants:** Cinnamon and apples are both high in antioxidants, which promote general health.
➢ **Tips:**
➢ **Optional:** Before baking, put chopped walnuts or almonds on top.
➢ **Make It Ahead:** Bake and reheat the apples before serving.
➢ **Pair with Spices:** Try adding ground ginger or cardamom for added flavor.

Chocolate-Dipped Strawberries

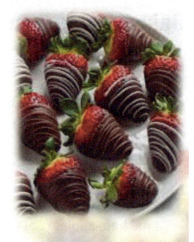

Prep Time: 10 minutes.
Cook Time: 5 minutes
Total Time: fifteen minutes
Serving Size: 4 (3 strawberries per serving)

Ingredients:

➢ 12 fresh strawberries.
➢ 1/4 cup unsweetened dark cocoa powder.
➢ 2 tablespoons water.
➢ 1/2 teaspoon of pure vanilla extract.
➢ Stevia or a zero-point sweetener (to taste)

Directions:

1. Prepare the Strawberries: - Wash and pat the strawberries dry, keeping the green top intact.

2. Prepare the Chocolate Dip: In a small saucepan, combine cocoa powder, water, vanilla essence, and sweetener. Cook over low heat, stirring regularly, until smooth and shiny.

3. Dip the Strawberries: Dip each strawberry by the green top into the chocolate sauce, covering approximately two-thirds of the berry. Place on a parchment-lined baking sheet.

4. Chill: Refrigerate the dipped strawberries for 10 minutes or until the chocolate is set.

5. Serve: Place strawberries on a dish and serve chilled.

Health Benefits:

➢ **Low in Calories:** Strawberries are naturally low in calories and high in water.
➢ **Rich in Antioxidants:** Both chocolate and strawberries are high in antioxidants, which promote heart and skin health.
➢ **Sugar-Free Option:** This dessert is naturally sweetened, making it a diabetic-friendly option.

Tips:

➢ Optional toppings include crushed nuts, shredded coconut, or cinnamon.
➢ **Experiment with Fruit:** Dip various fruits, such as banana slices or orange segments.
➢ **Quick Serving Idea:** Make a small quantity for a simple, last-minute treat.

Both dishes are simple, tasty, and fit wonderfully with a zero-point lifestyle.

Lemon & Coconut Energy Balls

Prep Time: 15 minutes.
Cooking time: None
Total Time: fifteen minutes
Serving Size: 10 (1 ball per serving)

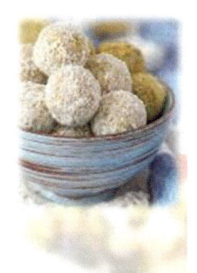

Ingredients:

➢ 1 cup unsweetened shredded coconut
➢ 1/2 cup almond flour (optional for texture; can be substituted with extra coconut for zero points).
➢ Zest from one large lemon.
➢ Juice from one huge lemon.
➢ Add 2 tbsp unsweetened applesauce and 1 tsp pure vanilla extract.
➢ Stevia or a zero-point sweetener (to taste)

Directions:

1. Prepare the Mixture: - In a mixing dish, combine the shredded coconut, almond flour (if using), lemon zest and juice, applesauce, vanilla essence, and sweetener. Mix until the ingredients combine into sticky dough.

2. Shape the Balls: - Scoop about a spoonful of the ingredients and roll it into a small ball with your palms. Repeat until all of the dough is used.

3. Chill: Place energy balls on a parchment-lined plate or tray and refrigerate for 30 minutes to firm up.

4. Serve: Store chilled in an airtight jar in the refrigerator for up to a week.

Health Benefits:

➢ **Energy Boost:** Coconut and lemon offer a natural energy boost without added sugar.
➢ **Rich in Healthy Fats:** Coconut contains healthy fats that will keep you satisfied.
➢ **Refreshing and Light:** Lemon provides a boost of vitamin C and a vibrant flavor.

Tips:

➢ **Customize the Flavor:** Add a pinch of turmeric or ginger for a unique taste.
➢ **Make It Extra Coconutty:** Roll the balls with more shredded coconut before cooling.
➢ **Freeze for Longer Storage:** These balls freeze well and can be consumed straight from the freezer.

Mango Sorbet

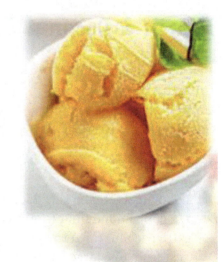

Prep Time: 5 minutes.
Freezing Time: 2 hours (for fresh mango)
Total time: 5 minutes (if using frozen mango).
Servings: 4

Ingredients:

➢ Three cups of frozen mango chunks
➢ Juice from 1 lime
➢ 1/4 cup water (or as required)

Directions:

1. In a high-speed blender or food processor, blend frozen mango pieces, lime juice, and water. Blend until smooth and creamy, adding water as required to get the right consistency.

2. To achieve a soft-serve texture, scoop the sorbet into dishes and serve immediately.

3. Freeze for Later: For a firmer texture, put the sorbet in a container and freeze for a further 1-2 hours before serving.

Health Benefits:

➢ **Rich in Vitamins**: Mango contains vitamins C and A and fiber.
➢ **Naturally Sweetened:** Mango's natural sweetness avoids the need for additional sugar.
➢ **Low Calories:** This dessert is light, guilt-free, and ideal for weight loss.

Tips:

➢ **Add Garnish:** For added flair, garnish with a sprig of mint or shredded coconut.
➢ **Experiment with Fruit:** For added diversity, substitute mango with pineapple or a combination of tropical fruits.
➢ **Make popsicles:** Pour the mixture into Popsicle molds and freeze for an enjoyable summer treat.

Both recipes are easy, delicious, and ideal for a healthier, zero-point lifestyle.

CONCLUSION

Reflections on Your Zero Point Journey

Congratulations on taking the initial steps toward adopting a better and more sustainable lifestyle with the Zero Point Approach! By taking this route, you've committed to feeding your body nutritious, nutrient-dense foods without the continual stress of counting calories or tracking every mouthful. This journey is about more than just losing weight; it's about developing a positive connection with food, improving your general health, and experiencing the joys of mindful eating.

WHAT YOU HAVE LEARNED

Through this cookbook, you have explored:

➤ **Zero-Point Foods:** The cornerstone of your meals, providing flexibility and freedom with your dietary choices.
➤ **Diverse Recipes:** From full breakfasts to filling dinners, snacks, and desserts, you've seen how great zero-point eating can be.
➤ **Meal Planning and Prep:** Resources for being organized and consistent while enjoying a variety of meals.
➤ **Healthy Habits:** How to stay motivated and on track without feeling confined or deprived.

CELEBRATION OF SMALL WINS

Every step you take, no matter how tiny, represents a success. Perhaps you've perfected a new recipe, discovered a novel technique to eat more vegetables, or simply felt better in your body after a week of zero-point meals. Celebrate these accomplishments; they are the foundation of long-term success.

A Bigger Picture

Your zero-point eating journey is more of a way of life than a diet. This method allows you to concentrate on fuelling your body with natural, nutritious meals that give you energy and improve your health. It's a manner of eating that promotes not only weight management but also mental and emotional health.

Remember that this is not about perfection. It's natural to deviate from your plan or consume meals that aren't zero points. What is important is your capacity to return to a balanced, attentive mindset.

Looking Ahead Remember these crucial principles as you continue on this journey:

➤ **Adaptability:** Feel free to change recipes to fit your preferences or what you have on hand. Zero-point eating is adaptable and works best when it integrates effortlessly into your lifestyle.
➤ **Consistency over Perfection:** Success comes from developing long-term routines rather than following strict rules.
➤ **Community and Support:** Share your experiences with friends, family, and others who are on the same road. Support and encouragement can make a significant difference.

A NEW RELATIONSHIP WITH FOOD

You've probably noticed a change in your attitude about food. It is no longer a cause of guilt or concern, but rather an occasion to rejoice and enjoy. You've learned to pay attention to your body's cues, fuel it with care, and indulge in moderation.

Final thoughts

The Zero Point journey is about more than just recipes; it's about adopting a new way of life. It's about waking up each day knowing you're making decisions that respect your body and help you achieve your goals. It's about enjoying the process, trying new flavors, and appreciating the variety of nutritional options available to you.

As you progress, remember that this is your journey, and you have the ability to mold it. Take the lessons you've learned from this cookbook and apply them in real life. Use the tools, advice, and recipes as a starting point for a healthier, happier you.

Here's to a lifetime of tasty, zero-point meals and satisfying, health-conscious living. The greatest is still to come!

Adjusting Recipes to Your Taste

One of the most powerful features of cooking is the option to customize recipes to your liking. While the recipes in this cookbook are intended to be delicious and healthful, they are also adaptable enough to meet your own tastes, dietary requirements, and imagination. Adapting recipes not only makes meals more delightful, but it also allows you to form a stronger connection with your food.

WHY ADAPT RECIPES?

➤ **Personal Preferences:** You may favor specific flavors, textures, or ingredients over others.
➤ **Dietary Restrictions:** Allergies, intolerances, or special dietary goals may necessitate modifications.
➤ **Seasonal Availability**: Fresh, local ingredients typically taste better and are less expensive.
➤ **Experimentation:** Trying different taste combinations can make cooking more interesting and enjoyable.

TIP FOR ADAPTING RECIPES

1. Make wise substitutions.

➤ **Replace proteins:** For a plant-based alternative, use turkey for chicken or tofu for beans.
➤ **Change the vegetables:** If a dish calls for zucchini but you prefer broccoli, make the substitution.
➤ **Experiment with grains**: For example, instead of quinoa, try farro, brown rice, or cauliflower rice.

2. Adjust seasonings to taste.

For an extra blast of flavor, add fresh herbs or citrus zest.

3. Experiment with cooking methods to suit your preferences, such as grilling instead of baking or steaming instead of sautéing.

4. **Portion Adjustments:** Scale recipes up or down to meet your needs. Preparing smaller or larger amounts minimizes waste and matches with your food plan.

5. **Cultural Fusion:** Incorporate tastes from your heritage or favorite cuisines. For example, use soy sauce in a vegetable stir-fry or curry powder in lentil recipes.

6. **Sweeten Naturally:** Use natural sweeteners like honey, maple syrup, or stevia instead of sugar. Tailor the sweetness levels in desserts or smoothies to your preferences.

7. **For richness, substitute plain Greek yogurt, avocado, or coconut milk for heavy cream. Alternatively, make it lighter.**
Reduce the use of oils and fats in lighter recipes and instead use broth or water.

PRACTICAL EXAMPLES

Breakfast Scramble: If preferred, add bell peppers or substitute spinach for kale.
Grilled Salmon: For a fresh variation, try a lime-cilantro marinade instead of lemon-garlic.
Lentil and Spinach Curry: Add more veggies like carrots or squash for texture.
Berry Parfait: To add diversity, try alternative fruits such as mango or kiwi.

REMAINING TRUE TO ZERO POINTS
When modifying recipes, remember to prioritize zero-point components such as fresh veggies, lean proteins, and fruits. This ensures that your reduced meals remain consistent with your weight loss goals.

FOSTERING CREATIVITY
Do not be frightened to experiment. Cooking is an art, and each change presents an opportunity to learn. Keep track of what works and what doesn't, and over time, you'll build a customized library of go-to recipes that are entirely your own.

Last Thoughts
Adapting recipes to your preferences means making your meals work for you. It's about celebrating the freedom and flexibility of cooking while prioritizing health and fitness. With a little imagination and confidence, every meal can be a delicious representation of your unique style and flavor preferences.

Tips for Long-Term Success

Starting a healthier lifestyle with the Zero Point approach is a huge step forward, but staying on track requires dedication, adaptability, and a positive attitude. The following advice will assist you in maintaining your success and incorporating this lifestyle into your daily routine.

FOCUS ON PROGRESS, NOT PERFECTION

➤ **Embrace Tiny Wins:** Celebrate every healthy choice, no matter how tiny.
➤ **Let Go of Guilt:** If you deviate from your goal, do not concentrate on it. Learn from the experience and move on.
➤ **Consistency over Perfection:** Long-term success is achieved by sticking to your goals most of the time, rather than striving for perfection.

PRIORITIZE MEAL PLANNING AND PREPARATION

➤ **Plan Ahead:** Schedule time each week to plan meals, shop for groceries, and prepare ingredients. **Batch cook:** Prepare meals in bulk and freeze portions for easy, zero-point options on busy days. **Stay stocked:** Keep your kitchen stocked with zero-point foods such as fresh veggies, lean proteins, and nutritious snacks.

KEEP THINGS INTERESTING

➤ **Try New Recipes:** Experiment with new recipes to keep meals lively and avoid boredom.
➤ **Experiment with Flavors:** Use herbs, spices, and condiments to create diversity without adding calories.
➤ **Rotate Ingredients:** Replace veggies, meats, or grains in meals to keep them fresh and in line with seasonal availability.

CREATE A SUPPORT SYSTEM

➤ **Involve Friends and Family:** Share your journey with loved ones for encouragement and support.
➤ **Join A Community:** Connect with others who have similar goals, whether online or in person, to share tips, recipes, and motivation.
➤ **Be Accountable:** Stay on track by sharing your progress and challenges with a trusted friend or group.

PRACTICE MINDFUL EATING

➤ **Slow Down:** Enjoy your meals and listen to your body's hunger and fullness cues.
➤ **Avoid distractions:** To really appreciate your cuisine, avoid using screens or multitasking while eating.
➤ **Portion Awareness:** To avoid overeating, use proper portions, including zero-point meals.

ADAPT TO LIFE'S CHALLENGES

➤ **Stay Flexible:** Accept that life's circumstances can change. Adjust your strategy as needed without sacrificing your aims.
➤ **Prepare for Special Events:** Make attentive choices and allow for moderate indulgences when navigating holidays, parties, and travel.
➤ **Bounce Back Quickly:** Don't allow an off day to disrupt your development. Refocus on your upcoming meal or activity.

MONITOR PROGRESS, including non-scale victories. Pay attention to increases in energy, mood, and fitness, not just weight.

➤ **Reflect regularly:** Take the time to assess what's working and where you can make improvements.
➤ **Create Realistic Goals:** Break down larger ambitions into manageable milestones to stay motivated.

PRIORITIZE SELF-CARE: GET enough rest to assist your body's recuperation and metabolism.
Remain Active: Include regular exercise in your regimen, even if it is simply a daily walk.
Reduce Stress: Use stress-management strategies such as meditation, yoga, or deep breathing to avoid emotional eating.

CONTINUOUS LEARNING

➤ **Educate Yourself:** Read books, articles, or attend workshops to learn more about nutrition and good practices.
➤ **Experiment:** Be willing to try different meals, cuisines, and cooking techniques to extend your horizons.

BE PATIENT WITH YOURSELF

➤ **Accept Setbacks:** Understand that progress is not always linear. Allow yourself grace at difficult times.
➤ **Celebrate Growth:** Recognize how far you've come, even if you're still working on your ultimate goals.

Last Thoughts

Long-term success is developing a sustainable lifestyle that works for you. It's a journey of discovering, adjusting, and developing your healthiest and happiest self. By incorporating these strategies into your daily routine, you will not only maintain your success but also thrive on your Zero Point journey. Remember that consistency, flexibility, and a positive outlook are essential for success—so continue to move forward with confidence!

Embracing a Healthier and Happier You

The route to a healthier, happier you is about more than simply what you eat or how much weight you lose; it's about changing your thinking, behaviours, and general approach to life. By adopting the Zero Point lifestyle, you've made an important step toward living with purpose and balance. This part is a meditation on what it means to fully accept and enjoy the colorful life you've worked so hard to build.

CELEBRATE YOUR PROGRESS

➤ **Recognize Your Achievements:** Recognize your accomplishments, such as trying new recipes, maintaining consistency, or meeting weight-loss targets.
➤ **Celebrate Non-Scale Victories:** Acknowledge gains in your energy, mood, confidence, and overall well-being.

CULTIVATE A POSITIVE MINDSET

➤ **Shift the Narrative**: Instead of focusing on what you're giving up, enjoy the abundance of delicious and nourishing options accessible.
➤ **Practice Gratitude:** Be grateful for your body and the attention you're providing it through mindful eating and exercise.
➤ **Be kind to yourself**: Accept that no road is perfect, and be compassionate to yourself amid failures.

MAINTAIN A BALANCED APPROACH

➤ **Find Your Rhythm:** Adopt a sustainable and enjoyable lifestyle, rather than one that is restrictive or stressful.
➤ **Allow for Indulgences:** Enjoy your favorite sweets on occasion without feeling guilty, remembering that balance is important.
➤ **Develop Healthy Rituals:** Incorporate enjoyable habits, such as weekly meal preparation, a morning smoothie regimen, or an evening walk.

CONNECT WITH YOUR FOOD

➤ **Understand Its Power:** Food provides fuel, medicine, and happiness. By eating nutrient-dense, zero-point meals, you're giving your body what it requires to thrive.
➤ **Cook with Intention**: Cooking should be viewed as a form of self-care and creativity, not a chore.
➤ **Enjoy the process:** Take time to appreciate the flavors, textures, and colors of your meals—it's a sensory experience that improves your overall well-being.

BUILD MEANINGFUL CONNECTIONS

➤ **Share Your Journey:** Encourage friends and family to join you in adopting better behaviors.
➤ **Cook Together:** Preparing meals with loved ones is a pleasant and fulfilling way to bond while also encouraging a shared commitment to health.

➢ **Inspire Others:** Your transformation may inspire individuals around you to make positive changes in their own lives.

KEEP GROWING

➢ **Stay Curious:** Try different recipes, cuisines, and culinary techniques to make your meals more fun and diversified.
➢ **Set new goals:** As you hit milestones, push yourself to new heights, whether it's mastering a challenging dish or adopting a new workout activity.
➢ **Adjust to Change:** Accept the natural evolution of your lifestyle when your preferences, needs, and circumstances shift.

EMBRACE JOY IN EVERYDAY LIFE:

➢ Focus on What Feels Good. Choose hobbies, foods, and habits that make you happy and reflect your ideals.
➢ **Celebrate Your Journey:** Health and pleasure are ongoing efforts, not final destinations. Enjoy each step of the journey.
➢ **Be present:** Live attentively, savoring the moments of delight, contentment, and fulfillment that come from nurturing your body and soul.

Last Thoughts

embracing a healthier, happier you entails much more than what's on your plate. It is a holistic journey that changes the way you live, think, and feel. Adopting the Zero Point lifestyle not only improves your physical health but also lays the groundwork for a happier and more balanced existence.

Remember that you are strong and deserve life's best. As you go, remember to nurture your body, foster happiness, and appreciate the vibrant, healthier version of yourself that you've worked so hard to achieve. Best wishes for a healthy, happy, and fulfilling life!

Stay Inspired

Staying inspired and motivated is essential for long-term success as you pursue health and wellness through the Zero Point lifestyle. It's simple to become distracted or lose focus, but with the correct materials and mindset, you can sustain your passion and keep going forward. The tactics listed below will keep you interested and excited about your goals while also providing next actions to help you grow and progress on this journey.

TRACK YOUR PROGRESS

Tracking your trip not only holds you accountable, but it also allows you to reflect on the progress you've made along the road.

➤ **Journaling:** Keep a dietary and exercise journal. Writing down your meals, workout routines, and thoughts might help you detect patterns, figure out what works, and stay focused on your objectives.
➤ **Photography:** Use images of your meals and activities to visually track your development. It's encouraging to see how far you've come, especially if you're feeling stuck.
➤ **Progress Report:** Evaluate your development every few weeks. How are you feeling, both physically and emotionally? Do you see any gains in your energy, mood, or overall health? Celebrate these achievements, regardless of their size.

TRY NEW ACTIVITIES AND FOODS

Variety makes things intriguing and eliminates boredom. To keep your routine interesting, try introducing new foods, physical activities, or cooking skills.

➤ **New Recipes:** Don't be scared to get out of your comfort zone. Try preparing dishes from new cultures or using things you've never cooked with before.
➤ **Fitness Adventures:** Swimming, cycling, yoga, and even hiking are all great ways to vary your routines.
➤ **Mindfulness activities:** Consider adding mindfulness activities like meditation, journaling, or yoga to improve both your mental and physical health.

REWARDING YOURSELF ALONG THE WAY

It is critical to acknowledge and reward your hard work. Treat yourself to small gestures that make you feel valued and driven.

➤ **Non-Food Rewards:** Purchase new exercise attire, take a relaxing bath, or pamper you with a spa day. Rewards should enhance your well-being rather than disrupt your progress.
➤ **Milestone Celebrations:** When you reach a key goal (for example, finishing 30 days on the Zero Point Diet), reward yourself with a special activity, such as going to the movies, attempting a new exercise class, or even taking a day off to relax and recharge.

REMEMBER YOUR "WHY"

As with any lifestyle adjustment, there will be days when you are unmotivated. On those days, it is critical to reconnect with your "why"—the reasons you began this journey in the first place.

➢ **Reflect on Your Purpose:** Whether you want to feel more energized, lose weight, or simply live a healthier life, remember the deep, personal reasons you started this path.

➢ **Visualize Your Future Self:** Consider how you will feel in a year—more confident, healthier, and full of life.

TAKE ACTION ON THE FOLLOWING STEPS

The adventure does not end with the final page of this cookbook. To stay on track for long-term success, focus on actionable next steps.

➢ **Weekly Meal Planning:** Set aside time each week to plan meals, prepare ingredients, and make sure you have everything you need to stay on track.

➢ **Incorporate New Habits:** Gradually introduce new habits into your routine, such as daily water, mindful eating, or 15 minutes of stretching.

➢ **Embrace Flexibility:** Life is unpredictable, so you must be adaptable. Don't be scared to change your strategy as needed while remaining focused on your aims.

Last Thoughts

staying inspired and motivated is a continuous process. It's normal to have peaks and troughs along the way, but with the appropriate skills, mindset, and resources, you'll stay on track to becoming a healthier, happier version of yourself. Accept each step of the path, enjoy tiny triumphs, and keep going forward with the assurance that you have all the power you need to reach your goals. Your success is not a destination; it is a lifelong journey!

Made in the USA
Coppell, TX
26 March 2025

47544645R00052